You have opened the cover of a book on a controversial subject. Perhaps you're just curious. If you are, the pages that follow will answer many of your questions. But if you, a close friend, or a member of your family has been affected by this frightening disease called AIDS, this handbook was written *expressly* for you. It can, and will, help you come to grips with the reality of AIDS, one step at a time, at your own pace.

Read at one sitting only what you can comfortably take in. Refer to the glossary to increase your understanding of medical terms. Share this book with your friends and family to open lines of communication and reassure your loved ones.

There is hope. Daily advances are made in understanding and treating the effects of this disease. And there is much you can do to make the quality of your life richer than it ever has been before. You are not alone. And you may have only begun to tap into the sources of strength you already possess that will give you the courage to live with AIDS.

It is the most positive resource I have seen for a person with HIV infection, and an absolute must for any person who is close to someone with AIDS. The next best thing to a personal psychotherapist.

—*Ivan B. John, M.D.*
Biotechnology consultant and volunteer physician
with the New York Community Health Project

There is no other book that so clearly addresses the problems of the patients with AIDS and their relationships with their families and friends.

—*Eskild A. Petersen, M.D.*
Chief of the Section of Infectious Diseases,
Department of Internal Medicine
at the University of Arizona Health Sciences Center

This book is exactly what I was looking for for my family. I did not know where to start. Even when I knew I could make it, nobody else saw it my way. Our family is using the book like a series of guideposts, and it really works. I know I'm going to make it, and I don't have to do it alone.

—*AIDS patient, New York*

Without this book our relationship would have fallen apart. I just knew it was over and I thought my life was finished. I was wrong. This book is fundamental: it offers real, honest, and positive approaches to important subjects. Since the day I found out I was HIV-positive, I've had two promotions at my job and bought a house. The book tells it like it is: It is possible to start over and live better.

—*AIDS patient, Phoenix*

Take These Broken Wings and Learn to Fly

The AIDS Support Book
for Patients, Family, and Friends

Steven D. Dietz and
M. Jane Parker Hicks, M.D.

Harbinger House
Tucson

The authors acknowledge with gratitude the following organizations:

National Institutes of Health, Bethesda, MD, for their kind permission
to freely adapt materials published by them.

Centers for Disease Control, Atlanta, GA, for generously providing slides
and materials on AIDS.

American Foundation for AIDS Research (AmFAR) for their
helpful resource guidance.

Harbinger House, Inc.
3131 North Country Club, Tucson, Arizona 85716
Printed in the United States of America
Set in 10/13 Linotron 202 Sabon.

Library of Congress Cataloging in Publication Data
Dietz, Steven D., 1947–
Take these broken wings and learn to fly : the AIDS support book for patients,
family, and friends / by Steven D. Dietz and M. Jane Parker Hicks.
p. cm.
Bibliography: p.
ISBN 0-943173-41-8 : $9.95
1. AIDS (Disease)—Handbooks, manuals, etc. 2. AIDS (Disease)—Psychological
aspects—Handbooks, manuals, etc. 3. AIDS (Disease)—Patients—
Rehabilitation—Handbooks, manuals, etc.
I. Hicks, M. Jane Parker, 1947–   . II. Title.
RC607.A26D54   1989   362.1'969792—dc20   89-7473

In loving memory of Steven,
the "King for a Day" who has found peace,
and in grateful appreciation of Robert,
whose joyful humor and zest for living
are a constant source of strength.

Contents

Contents

Introduction

"AIDS is an unbelievable motivation to stop procrastinating about doing the things we wanted to do—a reminder that past arguments we had aren't all that important after all. We take time now to love; there may not be another moment as great as the one right now for the two of us."

Those were the thoughts of a couple with AIDS who needed to share their feelings with someone who cared and who could understand.

We have written this handbook for those affected by AIDS: you, your family, someone you work with, someone you love. Our personal involvement, as professional care providers, has made us acutely aware of the anguish and the loneliness so many with AIDS have experienced and of the common bond that unites all who provide loving care for them. We feel equally the responsibility to share the understanding, faith, and courage with which our patients live their lives.

We have drawn, first and foremost, on letters, conversations, books and articles from, with, and by AIDS patients and their families and friends. In addition to publications by the Centers for Disease Control, the Public Health Service, and the World Health

Organization, we have learned much from the observations of professional colleagues working directly with the issues of AIDS. Our main emphasis, however, has been on the people who live with AIDS in their own lives: what they think, how they feel and what they do to cope with the disease.

For the sake of brevity, we have sometimes referred to persons with AIDS as though everyone infected with the Human Immunodeficiency Virus (HIV) fit in this category. That is most definitely not the case. If you have tested positive for antibodies, but show no signs of immune system impairment, you may not experience illness for a very long time—or at all. If, however, you have been diagnosed with AIDS, your tests show immune system impairment and you may already have suffered from a variety of opportunistic infections. These two physical conditions are critically different. Even so, the emotional trauma and resultant periods of psychological crisis can be nearly identical, whether or not there has been an actual diagnosis of AIDS. Knowing the facts about the road travelled by others can greatly reduce the stress for you—at any stage of infection or illness.

No two people with AIDS are alike, as are no two relatives or friends of people with AIDS. Although the material in this handbook is intended to be as universal as possible, some sections may not apply to your particular circumstances; other sections may make you feel uncomfortable. Each person has to cope with AIDS in an individual way. What follows is intended as a guide: a brief look at how some people with AIDS and their loved ones feel and the ways they found to deal with those feelings.

Although formal research on AIDS, its related diseases (also known as ARC or AIDS Related Complex), and treatment programs is limited, due to the relatively short time since the discovery of the disease, a great deal has been written on many of the subjects discussed in this book. If you desire more information, we strongly encourage you to make use of our list of recommended readings.

Any discussion of the Human Immunodeficiency Virus and the effects of HIV infection should begin with some background information about viruses, the concept of infection—with or without symptoms—and the immune system. We have included this in chapter 2. In addition, because of the sensitive nature of an infection that is sexually transmitted *and* potentially fatal, we have raised the issues of confidentiality, ethics, and legal implications throughout the book, wherever they apply.

The psychological impact of this infection reaches far beyond just those who are or will become infected. Disrupted family relationships can deeply alter the lives of those who never personally experience the disease. The loss of a beloved friend forever changes our concept of personal mortality. Anxiety about AIDS also cripples many who, for whatever reason, live in daily fear of potential infection. It is vital that, whatever your personal situation, you use this handbook only when you feel able to cope with the problems involved. Your emotions will tell you what pertains to you, and what you can grasp each day.

People with AIDS, close friends, and family members all face intense emotions that may be new to you. Only by exploring your emotions, a side of AIDS that neither surgery, drugs, nor diet can treat, can you dispel some of your feelings of fear, inadequacy, and loss of control over your future. You travel a road paved with an awesome mixture of hope and despair, courage and fear, humor and anger, and constant uncertainty. Sharing the experiences of others who have walked that road before will help you define your own feelings and find your own ways of coping.

It will help you keep your body strong if you also deal successfully with the emotional turmoil of AIDS. We will discuss some of the emotional problems you may face and some possible adjustments. We'll explore learning to express and share your feelings about AIDS, dealing with new responsibilities, coping with rejection by others, finding new meaning in your activities, and using each day to its fullest potential.

We all have good reason to identify, and learn to live with, our personal feelings about AIDS. AIDS is undeniably a major illness; it is often, though not necessarily, fatal and it may be with us for a long time. Today, nearly 1.5 to 2 million Americans are alive who have probably been infected with the Human Immunodeficiency Virus.

Eight years or more after initial HIV infection, one half of them may need treatment for the diseases related to AIDS.

For those who are already infected with HIV, as research continues, and newer, more reliable therapies are developed, AIDS may well become just another chronic condition, treatable in much the same way as rheumatoid arthritis, diabetes, or emphysema. Just as for patients with other chronic conditions, periodic health checkups will be part of the lifelong routine of those infected with HIV. And, although they will be more sensitive to, and anxious about, minor signs of illness or discomfort, they most likely will need their lifelong medication or special diets to remind them each day that they have been infected with a virus that was once considered deadly. Many will live for years, and some will grow old and die much as they had expected to do before AIDS was recognized. Some may never experience AIDS-related illness, but will live with physical examinations and blood tests that serve as constant reminders of potential immune deficiency.

There are normal phases of emotional response that everyone touched by this disease goes through: shock, anger, denial, depression, grief, and attempts at "bargaining for answers." We have written this book to help you take control of emotional instability and move *through* these phases, into a hopeful and productive future.

At the moment your HIV test is confirmed positive, you may find it difficult not to dwell on thoughts of dying, but it is vitally important that you focus instead on living. Remember, testing positive for HIV infection is not an imminent death sentence! Many of the related conditions common to AIDS can now be treated. Patients with more serious infections may live long enough to benefit from treatments yet to be discovered.

Indeed, there are sunrises as well as sunsets to be enjoyed. You can set aside doubts about the quantity of your days and begin to improve the quality of your life—a life touched by AIDS and its treatment, but yours to sense, feel, and live nonetheless.

Chapter 1

Searching for Explanations

"Don't let us make imaginary evils,
when you know we have so many real ones to encounter."
OLIVER GOLDSMITH

By the time Goldsmith wrote those words, the plague had ravaged Europe for centuries. Few examples so clearly show the destructive side of the human imagination. Ignorance about the disease was nearly universal; misconceptions and irrational conclusions born of fear became almost as great a threat to life as the plague itself.

When faced with life-threatening personal crisis, you experience a natural mental progression that can take you from intense fear and apprehension, to unrelenting self-examination, to a sense of guilt that eats away at your self-image. If you can't find the answers you seek, you may begin to draw your own negative conclusions. The common belief that only the "bad" are prone to serious illness is one such "conclusion" that will endanger your mental health.

Just as the plague was the result of a bacterium, and not evil witchcraft, HIV infection is the result of a virus, and not the punishment of a cruel spirit. HIV is a virus, an unfortunate development in biological evolution that has brought about devastating health problems, but a virus just the same.

Further complicating the issues of ill health, persons infected with the Human Immunodeficiency Virus and those suffering from full-blown AIDS must often confront a range of additional problems from discrimination and addictive behavior to the loss of privacy, self-reliance, and financial resources. Little wonder that so many feel the future is bleak and seek someone to blame. Tremendous credit is due those who, setting aside their fear and anger, bravely choose to pick up the pieces of their lives and face the future with a sense of purpose and hope.

For a time, following the discovery of the virus that causes AIDS, there was a sense of urgency to find the origin of the virus. Theories were as numerous as scientists seeking the source. Nations, organizations, racial groups, persons involved in homosexual or bisexual lifestyles, and users of intravenous drugs all shuddered as the finger of blame pointed in their direction. When scientists discovered the virus and realized that it knew no borders, nor was it selective by race, age, or sex, a new trend began in research to neutralize its effect on human life. Public policy made a notable shift. It became far more important to stop the spread of this new disease than to find its place of birth.

Still, on a personal level, we seek answers. Our natural curiosity wants to find the *reason* for all that has happened, and is happening, in our lives. "Whose fault is it? What did I do wrong?" It is as though placing blame will reverse the loss. Science may continue its search for the origin for many decades to come. But if you, or someone close to you, is facing the many issues of AIDS, it is time to begin a more productive focus on the essential facts. AIDS is biological. You did not come to this point because of errors of faith, nor good deeds left undone. You are not waging a predestined and hopeless battle with fate. Although the medical terms may seem confusing, your physical body is simply fighting infection.

Your friend, facing illness, does not need to be judged for behavior that may be different from your own. What he does need is your understanding, respect, and support as he faces the realities of what can and must be done today.

Early in the days of counseling cancer patients, it was not uncommon to hear the phrase "cancer victim." Every disease considered "incurable" or "chronic"; every event that brought about any unpredictable loss; and every "act of God" that brought about devastation came to be described with its own set of "victims." Those with courage and a strong sense of self-respect began to reject such indiscriminate labels. They were not as much "victims" as they were people who had been "unprepared at the moment of assault," but who, picking up the pieces of their lives, overcame their difficulties. To be defined as a "victim" too often implies permanent disability— that life will from that day forward be painfully restricted.

The use of labels may seem insignificant to the casual observer, but for people personally affected by serious disease, accurate descriptions that allow for hope, change, and legitimate progress are vital.

If you are now infected with HIV because of contaminated blood products that you did not suspect, sexual preferences that others do not accept, or intravenous drugs that have taken more control of your life than you planned, the last thing you need now is someone, however well-intentioned, pointing a finger at you. Seeking reasons from the past may well be the poorest use of your time, and all too often, you will end up pointing the finger at yourself.

Certainly there are occasions when, in order to correct unsuccessful behavior or attitudes, a therapist must assist you in unscrambling past events to make sense of present difficulties. Self-destructive behavior or repeated patterns of action that bring you pain need to be understood and changed. But far more frequently, what you need most at the moment of crisis is someone who can help you sort through the difficulties of "today"; someone who will help you step confidently out of the spiral of self-incrimination.

Even though you may feel almost hopelessly confused by the complex issues related to HIV infection, the starting point is extremely simple: you have a known viral infection and transmission of that infection is preventable.

Other have faced the emotional turmoil of AIDS before you. Still others will follow who will gain strength and determination from your example, and from those who help you on your path. Your first goal must be to move forward with purpose from this moment.

For now, we start at the beginning. What is this virus, how is it transmitted, and what challenges does it present you, your family, and friends?

Chapter 2

The Virus That Changes Life

What Is AIDS?

What is this disease that has so greatly changed our lives, created fear and anxiety, and led to one of the greatest medical research efforts of recent times? In May, 1987, the Centers for Disease Control defined AIDS as "the presence of a reliably-diagnosed disease that is at least moderately indicative of a problem of underlying cellular immune deficiency in people less than the age of 60 who have no other known causes of immune deficiency, are not on any immune suppressant therapy, and do not have a lymphoma or Hodgkin's disease, both known to be associated with immune suppression." This definition and subsequent revisions were designed to distinguish the newly recognized Acquired Immune Deficiency Syndrome (AIDS) from other previously recognized causes of acquired immune deficiency and to describe the syndrome in such a way that could be accurately studied as to its cause and means of transmission.

By 1984, it was becoming apparent that AIDS was caused by a virus and that, to some degree, it was contagious. To understand the importance of this discovery, and the results of infection with this new virus, some background information about the normal human immune system and the AIDS virus (HIV) is essential.

The Immune System

The immune system is a network of specialized cells, tissues and organs that extends throughout the body. Its main defenses are formed by white blood cells in the body's blood and lymph, chiefly by: polys (polymorphonuclear leukocytes), monocytes (also called macrophages in the tissues), and lymphocytes. All these cells originate in the bone marrow, the central portion of our bones and the source of all blood cells after birth. In addition, lymphocytes are found in the lymph nodes, scattered throughout the body, and in the spleen, the principal immune organ of the blood, which contains every kind of cell normally found in the blood and which is located in the lower left side of the rib cage. Also vital to the immune system is the thymus, a gland in the lower neck and upper chest that programs specialized lymphocytes called T-cells. The thymus shrinks and all but disappears by the time we are seven or eight years old, but it continues to secrete hormones that induce the formation of T-cells.

There are two major kinds of immune response: natural (or innate) and specialized (or acquired). Our first line of defense, the natural immune response, brings into action the polys and the monocytes-macrophages. These cells are "naturally" attracted to foreign matter, for example, a microbe or a splinter, which they engulf and digest. In fact, macrophage literally means "big eater." Most foreign invaders, e.g., microbes, are effectively destroyed by our natural immune response. To combat those which are not, a second line of defense, the specialized immune response, is normally activated, which mobilizes the lymphocytes.

There are two major types of lymphocytes: B-cells and T-cells. B-cells mature into plasma cells that destroy microbes in the blood and body fluids by means of a variety of antibodies. The B-cell immune response is also called the humoral immune response because the antibodies B-cells produce are soluble humors in the blood and body fluids. T-cells are specially programmed by the thymus. They are responsible for what is called the cellular immune response, because when first discovered, T-cells were thought to act directly—

as cells. One of their most important protective jobs is to kill virus-infected cells.

Some microbes, such as most bacteria, live a free existence (extracellular) in tissues or body fluids, while other, such as viruses, live inside cells (intracellular). B-cells and plasma cells use antibodies primarily to neutralize extracellular microbes, while T-cells act primarily against intracellular microbes.

T-cells are divided into two subtypes with widely differing functions: cytotoxic or killer T-cells, which directly destroy target cells, for example, virus-infected cells, and regulatory T-cells, which regulate the entire specialized immune system. Regulatory T-cells are further divided into helper T-cells and suppressor T-cells. As their names suggest, helper T-cells induce or help the functions of the specialized immune response—both the humoral (B-cell) and cellular (T-cell)—while suppressor T-cells down-regulate or suppress those same functions. If the immune system were not suppressed, or turned off, after it had removed or destroyed foreign microbes, it would begin to attack healthy tissue. This happens in some autoimmune diseases such as rheumatoid arthritis or lupus erythematosis, where the immune response is not adequately suppressed.

The helper T-cell is the single most important cell in the specialized immune system. Helper T-cells coordinate, or play an essential role in, both humoral and cellular immune responses. Through soluble substances called lymphokines, they activate or assist B-cells (and through B-cells, antibody production), killer T-cells, and macrophages. Because of the critical coordinating role of helper T-cells, the specialized immune response cannot function without them, and any defect in these cells will cripple the immune system as a whole.

Not everyone is born with an intact immune system. There are many inherited as well as acquired (not inherited) immune system defects. For example, some infants are born without T-cells because their thymus fails to develop. These infants have no T-cell immune response and develop a variety of infections that normally would not cause disease in healthy persons. And because the immune response is also important in preventing development of malignant tumors, there are other inherited forms of immune deficiency that are associated with an increased likelihood of certain types of cancers. It is believed that, at any given moment, we all have a few cells with the potential to become cancers, but if we also have healthy, functioning T-cells, the potential cancer cells are destroyed well before they can ever grow into tumors.

Immune deficiency syndromes have been recognized for many decades. In the early eighties, when the effects of HIV infection were first observed, it was obvious that the patients were suffering from an acquired (not inherited) form of immune deficiency that looked very much like a defect of the cellular immune (T-cell) response. Viruses had also been studied for decades and were known to cause a variety of diseases. Viral infection had even been recognized as the indirect cause of transient, mild immune deficiency. What had *not* been observed before the discovery of HIV was a virus that infected, and effectively destroyed, the single most important cell of the specialized immune response, the helper T-cell.

The "Backward" Virus

Viruses are submicroscopic particles, smaller than the individual cells that make up our tissues and organs. In contrast to most microbes, viruses are incomplete organisms: they cannot survive by themselves but must live inside other cells and can only reproduce inside other cells. They are composed of genetic material, DNA (deoxyribonucleic acid) *or* RNA (ribonucleic acid), proteins, and an outer covering. Normally, our cells contain inherited genes in the form of DNA. When cells in our body grow and divide, the DNA molecules act as templates that instruct the cell to produce RNA, which, in turn, acts to produce the proteins that accomplish most of the metabolic functions necessary for life. Therefore, the usual sequence of events is as follows: first, DNA is used to make RNA; then, RNA is used to make proteins.

Viruses that contain DNA use the infected (or host) cell's machinery to follow the same sequence as normal cells to produce RNA and the proteins necessary to form new viruses. Ordinarily, viruses that contain RNA form new viruses by producing protein directly from the RNA, skipping the initial DNA step.

In the early 1970's, among viruses that infect animals, a new type RNA virus was discovered. This type contained, along with its RNA, a unique enzyme called reverse transcriptase that enabled RNA to act as a template for DNA, instead of the other way around. Because of this "backward" step (RNA to DNA instead of DNA to RNA), these viruses are called retroviruses (retro = backwards). The DNA produced by the virus from its RNA is called a provirus and it becomes part of the infected cell's DNA. When the infected cell is stimulated to grow and reproduce, the virus-derived DNA is also stimulated to produce viral RNA and proteins, and thus more viruses as well.

Although not new in veterinary medicine, retroviruses were first found to cause disease in humans in 1979–1980 by Dr. Robert Gallo (National Cancer Institute, Bethesda, Maryland) and also by a group of Japanese investigators, who independently defined Human T-cell Leukemia-Lymphoma Virus Type 1 (HTLV-I). This first human lymphotropic retrovirus also infected helper T-cells, but instead of bringing on an obvious immune deficiency, it caused a malignancy of the helper T-cells that resulted in a cancer of the blood and bone marrow. Other organs of the lymphatic system that can become involved with malignancy are the lymph nodes (the glands in our neck or under our arms, which sometimes swell up when we are fighting off an infectious disease) and the spleen (an organ in the lower left side of the rib cage). Malignancies of lymphocytes in the lymph nodes and spleen are called lymphomas. Eventually, two viruses were found to be associated with malignancies of lymphocytes, HTLV-I and HTLV-II.

Then, in 1983, Luc Montagnier and a group of his coworkers from the Pasteur Institute in Paris reported their discovery of an altogether new virus. They took a lymph node from a patient with the AIDS-related lymphadenopathy syndrome (enlarged lymph nodes, fever, and unusual weight loss), and cultured a virus they called Lymphadenopathy-Associated Virus or LAV. The virus turned out to be a retrovirus. Dr. Robert Gallo, a well-known expert in retrovirology, and his coworkers in Bethesda, Maryland, were able to isolate a similar virus from AIDS patients in the United States. Finally in April, 1984, Dr. Gallo reported the discovery of a virus he called Human T-cell Lymphotropic Virus Type III (HTLV-III). Because of its unique effects upon the human immune system, it was eventually renamed Human Immunodeficiency Virus (HIV).

When this virus was discovered, it was already known that transient, mild immune deficiency could follow a viral infection, for example, measles or infectious mononucleosis. And retroviruses themselves had been previously recognized as causes of human disease. What was unique about HIV infection was that the virus *directly* attacked the single most important cell responsible for activating and coordinating the specialized immune response, the helper T-cell. By attacking this cell, HIV infection leads to an acquired (rather than inherited) immune deficiency that severely weakens and may destroy the body's defense against infection, even against microbes that ordinarily do not cause disease, such as *Pneumocystis carinii,* and against uncommon malignancies, such as Kaposi's sarcoma. An infection caused by microbes that usually do not produce disease is called an opportunistic infection.

HIV and the Immune System

The lymphocytes mentioned above, helper T-cells and suppressor-killer T-cells, are identified by unique molecules or markers on their surfaces, labeled in this case CD4 (or T4) and CD8 (or T8) respectively. These surface molecules are essential for the normal functioning of T-cells, and hence for the normal functioning of the T-cell immune response. The CD4 molecule acts as a cell surface receptor for HIV, enabling the virus to enter directly into a living cell.

Normally, healthy people have twice as many helper T-cells in their bloodstream as they have suppressor-killer T-cells. Therefore the helper-to-suppressor ratio (as it is commonly called) is approximately 2 to 1 (2:1). Usually, there are more than 1,000 helper T-cells per microliter of blood (500 is the lower limit of normal), and more than 500 suppressor-killer T-cells per microliter of blood (300 to 1,100 per microliter is the normal range). Sophisticated chemical markers (monoclonal antibodies) are used to identify the different lymphocytes and classify them into different categories: helper or suppressor-killer T-cells. (Standard laboratory methods cannot distinguish between suppressor T-cells and killer T-cells.)

Soon after HIV infection, the immune system may appear to be functioning normally because the patient shows no signs of disease, and indeed, T-cell numbers may be normal. However, later testing usually reveals a decrease in the number of helper T-cells. When this happens, the helper-to-suppressor ratio falls, often to very low levels: from the normal 2:1 to 1:2 (0.5), or even lower. But it is important to understand that the helper-to-suppressor ratio may be low for any of three reasons:

1. a decrease in the number of helper T-cells;
2. an increase in the number of suppressor-killer T-cells; or
3. a combination of both (1) and (2).

All of the above may occur as a result of HIV infection. At different stages of infection and in different patients the levels of T-cells can be affected in different ways. Because HIV attacks helper T-cells, a low ratio due to a decrease in the number of helper T-cells strongly suggests HIV infection. But, early in HIV infection, the ratio may be low for another reason: the number of helper T-cells may still be normal, while the number of suppressor-killer T-cells is elevated in response to the infection. However, because this combination (normal level of helper T-cells, high level of suppressor-killer T-cells) also occurs in many other infectious diseases, a low ratio due to an increase in suppressor-killer T-cells is *not* specific for HIV infection.

Much still needs to be known about why these different changes in T-cell levels occur. What is apparent is that decreasing numbers of helper T-cells are associated with actively progressing disease and that very high levels of suppressor-killer T-cells (greater than about 1200 per microliter) suggest a high likelihood of disease progression within a few years.

Individuals infected with *Pneumocystis carinii* (opportunistic pneumonia infection) usually have very low levels of helper T-cells (generally 200 or less per microliter) and low helper-to-suppressor ratios (1:2 or less). Those developing Kaposi's sarcoma or lymph node malignancies (lymphomas) often have higher ratios (approximately 1:1). Remember, the ratio in healthy individuals is 2:1 or higher.

The Role of Antibodies in HIV Infection

Don't antibodies protect us from diseases? In some cases, that certainly is true. Once we've had hepatitis B, for example, antibodies protect us from getting that type of hepatitis B again.

A different situation exists with Herpes simplex, the virus that causes cold sores or fever blisters. Many of us have been exposed to this virus and have developed antibodies to it by the time we are teenagers. However, these antibodies do not protect us from getting cold sores from time to time throughout our lives.

Herpes simplex and related viruses reproduce their genetic material inside the host cell's DNA, where it lies dormant or latent, probably for the life of the cell—in this case a nerve cell. Because antibodies cannot reach inside the cell to the DNA where the virus resides, they are not effective in eliminating the virus from the body, or in preventing the recurrence of cold sores. By some unknown mechanism, physical or mental stress stimulates the viral DNA in the host cell to produce more Herpes viruses, and a cold sore develops.

Like Herpes simplex, HIV makes viral DNA part of the infected cell's DNA, where it remains dormant, probably for the life of the cell, and where it cannot be reached by antibodies. Also like Herpes simplex, dormant HIV needs a stimulus, such as another infection, to trigger production of more HIV, but there the similarity ends. Unlike Herpes simplex, the activated HIV attacks and directly infects the most important cell (helper T-cell) of the specialized immune response; destruction of these cells brings about a severe immune deficiency.

At this time, many different types of HIV antibodies have been discovered, some of which may play a role in protecting us from active HIV infection (when the virus is being made and released from the infected cells). But for now at least, the presence of antibodies serves primarily as a marker that HIV has entered the body—that HIV infection has occurred—and that the specialized immune response has been activated. Testing for HIV antibodies is therefore the primary diagnostic tool in determining HIV infection. A person with HIV antibodies is called seropositive for HIV.

What Is HIV Infection?

When HIV infects the helper T-cells, three results may occur: asymptomatic infection, AIDS-Related Complex (ARC), or AIDS itself. These three results usually represent different phases of the disease. But do they always? This is one of the unanswered questions concerning HIV infection.

HIV infection may take different forms in different persons. These variations will be discussed below, but first, it is extremely important to understand the concept of asymptomatic infection. Infection is defined as the entry of a microbe (in this case, a virus) into a susceptible living cell. Often, when a virus enters a cell and influences the host cell to produce additional viruses, there is no adverse effect on the host. In other words, no symptoms or disease. This is called asymptomatic infection, and it is a common form of infection. Asymptomatic infection is often a difficult concept to understand because of our tendency to equate infection with illness or disease. But remember the last time everyone around you had a cold, and you didn't get sick? You may have been asymptomatically infected.

When a virus enters a susceptible cell and makes itself part of the genetic material of the infected cell, without necessarily producing more viruses, it is called silent or latent infection. As mentioned earlier, many viruses do this, including the Herpes family of viruses, which cause cold sores (or fever blisters), genital ulcers, and infectious mononucleosis (sometimes called the kissing disease). These viruses may remain inside their hosts for life, with only an occasional cold sore or genital lesion to show for it. The majority of humans (probably over 80%) have been infected with these viruses and are living comfortably with them.

The human retrovirus HIV exhibits similar characteristics. Following infection or entry of the virus into helper T-cells, there may or may not be a recognizable, brief episode of fever, fatigue, and swollen lymph nodes. Then the virus enters the genetic material of the infected cell and resides there in a dormant or latent state. Individuals with asymptomatic infection exhibit no symptoms but are in effect "carriers" of the disease because their systems contain intermittent low levels of virus produced by infected cells. Following a period of time ranging from months to years, greater numbers of infected T-cells begin to produce greater numbers of virus and, in effect, the virus becomes activated. It is unknown at this time exactly what proportion of individuals latently infected with HIV will ultimately progress to active infection, but the most recent evidence indicates that it takes an average of eight years to progress from initial HIV infection through the latent phase (incubation period) to full-blown AIDS.

Active infection can then take on a variety of forms, often referred to as AIDS-Related Complex (ARC). ARC symptoms may include persistent fever, night sweats, unintentional weight loss, fatigue, swollen lymph nodes, oral thrush (a yeast infection), chronic diarrhea, and in some cases, serious, long-term occurrences of psoriasis or shingles. About 20%–50% of the people that have tested HIV-seropositive have thus far developed ARC. The most dangerous form of HIV infection is full-blown AIDS, characterized by several types of serious infections and cancers (including Kaposi's sarcoma and lymphoma) that are life-threatening.

HIV infection may show different patterns of progression. The most common has already been described: an initial non-specific flu-like illness, followed by a long-term latent period of no symptoms and low levels of virus production and finally by more active infection with higher levels of virus production. The number of helper

T-cells is usually low during the latent phase, but during the later, activated stage of infection this number may decrease dramatically. Antibodies to HIV are usually present within six to eight weeks of infection and usually stay detectable throughout the illness, although antibody levels may decrease very late in the disease. Virus components may actually be detected as early as two weeks after infection, persisting for two to four months, and then reappearing in the later stages of disease, as antibody levels decrease.

Another pattern of infection begins with acute illness, followed by a latent, asymptomatic phase, as described above. In a few of these infected individuals there is no evidence of virus production and HIV antibody levels are negative or undetectable. It is possible that more sensitive methods may be developed that will detect evidence of virus. The significance of these findings is uncertain, but these individuals may have controlled the infection. Long-term follow up is needed to determine whether or not these persons have truly controlled the infection.

Finally, there are indivduals who are infected but who show detectable evidence of HIV antibody or virus only after many months, and then at very low levels. Again, we need to wait several more years to learn how infections following this pattern ultimately progress. However, the mere fact that there are different ways of responding to this infection is a source of great optimism.

Where Is the Virus?

As mentioned previously, HIV infects, and thus is found within, the helper T-cells. In addition, HIV may also infect B-cells and other lymphocytes, monocytes and macrophages, and many other blood and body cells that may or may not express the CD4 molecule on their surface. The virus is therefore found in the blood, in the bone marrow, where the blood is made, and in the lymph nodes, where the lymphocytes reside. HIV has also been found in cells of the brain and intestine.

The virus can also be found briefly *outside* blood cells in the plasma (the liquid portion of the blood). This explains why hemo-philiacs have been infected in the past with contaminated plasma products used to treat their blood-clotting disorders. The virus has been isolated from saliva, urine, semen, vaginal and cervical secre-tions, and tears.

It is important to realize that the presence of detectable virus in a body fluid does *not prove* that the virus can be *transmitted* by exposure to that fluid. How the disease is *actually* transmitted will be discussed below.

How HIV Is Transmitted

HIV IS TRANSMITTED BY KNOWN ROUTES.
INFECTION IS ALWAYS THE RESULT OF THE EXCHANGE
OF BODY FLUIDS.
IT IS TRANSMITTED BY INTIMATE SEXUAL CONTACT
WITH EXCHANGE OF GENITAL SECRETIONS,
BY CONTAMINATED BLOOD AND BLOOD PRODUCTS,
AND FROM A MOTHER TO HER INFANT.

It is important to understand that medical science determines how an infectious disease is transmitted by *direct* observation of *actual* cases. The study of disease transmission is the subject of epidemiology, and there are well-established and proven methods to determine exactly how diseases are spread from person to person within a population.

Sexual transmission of HIV occurs with the exchange of body fluids, including semen and vaginal secretions. It is the actual entry of fluids containing infected cells into our bodies (blood, semen, vaginal secretions) that causes infection. The presence of genital sores or ulcers appears to increase the likelihood of disease transmis-sion by making it easier for infectious fluids to enter the body through breaks in the skin or lining of the genital tract. Breaks in the lining of the anus or rectum would also facilitate sexual transmission by receptive anal intercourse.

Transmission of HIV by contaminated blood occurs in several ways. The most direct way is through transfusion of blood from an infected donor. This is a rare occurrence today because all blood for transfusion is tested for HIV. However, the test is not perfect. Therefore, persons from groups at high risk for infection are screened out as blood donors, and doctors are exercising greater caution in the use of blood transfusions. In the case of hemophiliacs, exposure has come from the use of contaminated factor VIII (a blood-clotting product made from blood). Because this product is now prepared in a way that destroys HIV, transmission by this route will become very rare. Finally, intravenous drug users who share needles may be exposed when they inject, along with the drug, contaminated blood remaining in the syringe from the prior, infected user. In all these instances, it's blood or fluid to bloodstream that transmits infection.

An infant born to a mother with HIV infection is at high risk for becoming infected. During pregnancy and delivery there can be an exchange of blood between the baby and the mother. Also, during delivery the baby is exposed to contaminated secretions in the mother's genital tract. Newborn infants have relatively immature immune systems and are more susceptible, in general, to infection. Any one or all of these mechanisms may explain the observed transmission of infection from mother to newborn baby. In rare cases, caretakers of infants with AIDS have developed HIV infection. These infants often have severe, watery diarrhea, and exposure to large amounts of contaminated diarrhea is the presumed mode of transmission.

From observed cases of HIV transmission, high risk behaviors for contracting infection have been defined. These include: (1) unprotected sexual intercourse; (2) sharing of dirty intravenous needles; and (3) blood transfusion (this is a major problem in developing countries with a large number of AIDS cases, such as in Africa).

How HIV Is Not Transmitted

HIV infection is not easily transmitted. It is not transmitted by casual contact, for example, by touching, hugging, hand-shaking, drinking from the same glass, using the same eating utensils, or sharing a toilet seat or water fountain. Where there has been no high risk behavior, household contacts of persons with AIDS have simply *not* been infected.

Considerable attention has been given to the presence of HIV in saliva, and much theoretical concern has been voiced about the possibility that kissing, especially "deep" kissing, might transmit the infection. There has, however, been no evidence that saliva or kissing can transmit the disease. Indeed, when all other known routes of transmission (for example, sexual intercourse) of HIV infection have been ruled out, there have been *no* cases of HIV infection transmitted by saliva or kissing. From a common sense point of view, if HIV were transmitted by saliva, no amount of underreporting of AIDS cases could mask the full-scale epidemic that would have resulted.

And finally, there is no evidence that even mosquito bites transmit HIV infection.

Opportunistic Infections

Opportunistic infections are caused by organisms which do not ordinarily cause disease in persons with healthy immune systems, but to which most of us have been exposed at some time in our lives. For example, *Pneumocystis carinii* is a single-celled organism to which about 90% of us have antibodies by the time we are four years old, meaning we have been exposed to this organism as children. *Pneumocystis carinii* does not cause pneumonia in people whose immune systems are intact. Only when the immune system is seriously impaired, as with active HIV infection, do these organisms have the "opportunity" to cause infection. Such infections are therefore called opportunistic infections. Doctors are more familiar with these infections from treating them in cancer patients who have undergone intensive chemotherapy, a non-infectious cause of acquired immune deficiency.

Infections That Change Diagnosis

In resource literature the term ARC or AIDS-Related Complex is used to include a wide variety of associated diseases observed in

HIV-infected persons, but *not* included in the CDC's strict definition of AIDS (which was expanded and revised in September, 1987). Because scientists know that the diseases are related to AIDS, they refer to them under the term ARC.

Prior to the discovery of HIV as the cause of this disease, AIDS was often compared to hepatitis B, with respect both to the people (risk groups) infected, and to the mode of transmission. As with HIV, not everybody who gets infected with the hepatitis B virus has the same manifestations of infection. Some people infected with hepatitis B develop fulminant liver failure and die very quickly—like those at the tip of the AIDS iceberg. Some people get hepatitis and turn yellow; some people get hepatitis and *don't* turn yellow. Some become asymptomatic carriers, without ever knowing they have been infected, and some people have an effective immune response and become immune. With both hepatitis B and AIDS, the concept of a spectrum of responses to viral infection may explain why the same virus produces such different manifestations in the persons it infects.

The puzzles of manifestation are frustrating, but also a source of hope. Not knowing for certain how, or whether, the disease will progress may increase feelings of insecurity, but knowing that a few persons infected with the virus seem to have developed an immunity to it, or to have controlled its progression, reinforces the hope that full-blown AIDS may not occur in everyone infected with HIV. The fact that more opportunistic diseases are being successfully treated for longer periods also adds valuable time for research, and gives persons with AIDS an opportunity to take control of their own health—mental as well as physical.

Taking the Test

HIV testing is performed primarily for three reasons: to detect infection in an individual patient, to determine, by screening large numbers of people, how many are infected within a population (epidemiology), and to detect infected blood products and eliminate them from the blood supply. At the very outset, it is important to stress that *no laboratory test is perfect!* Inaccurate test results may arise from unusual but natural disease manifestations, from human error, or from technical error.

There is general agreement that HIV testing is needed to diagnose HIV infection in consenting individuals who appear to have AIDS or other conditions associated with HIV infection. There is also general agreement that testing is needed to screen various groups within the population to determine how many persons may be unknowingly transmitting the disease to others, and by what specific routes they are transmitting it. These two applications of testing are called diagnostic and epidemiologic testing. However, because of the stigma that has been attached to HIV infection, there still is much controversy about how to proceed with testing or screening for HIV.

The need to protect confidentiality has been widely debated. Some argue that total confidentiality can be achieved, even without anonymity, while others argue that confidentiality cannot be guaranteed in any setting. Our purpose here is not to address this controversy, but to encourage you to be certain of the protections available to you in safeguarding the privacy of your own medical records. Don't be afraid to ask about confidentiality. Find out what will be done with your test results, who will have access to them, and what guarantees are available, in writing if necessary.

The usual laboratory tests for HIV detect the presence of HIV antibodies and are called serologic tests. The initial test normally used is the ELISA or EIA. This test has a high sensitivity, which means that almost everyone with HIV infection will have a positive result. The trade-off for such high sensitivity is that some persons *without* disease will also test positive, producing what are called *false* positive test results. The initial test therefore "over-detects" infection. However, when the most important consideration is to detect *everyone* with disease infection, high sensitivity is essential. The long-term emotional cost of *missing* a diagnosis is greater than the short-term (usually no more than a week) emotional trauma caused by an initial false positive test. Within a week, all positive test results by the initial test should be *confirmed*—or overturned—by using a second test that almost always gives positive results only for

patients with HIV infection. These are called *true* positive test results. The confirmatory test normally used is the Western blot. This
illustrates the importance of educating patients about HIV testing.
All persons being tested need to be informed of the possibilities of
false positive test results.

You may ask why take the initial test at all. Although false
positive test results can occur, the vast majority (95% to 99%) of
test results are accurate. The initial test is easier to perform and costs
less.

The sequence of events normally followed for HIV testing is as
follows:

1. The patient's consent to test is obtained; the patient is
   counseled regarding the limitations of testing (for example,
   the potential for false positive results with the initial test);
2. The initial test is performed, and if the test result is negative,
   it is reported to the patient immediately;
3. If the initial test is positive or questionable (the answer is
   not always clear-cut), the same sample is repeated in *dupli-
   cate*. If both repeats are negative, the test is considered
   negative. If one or both repeats are positive, the test is
   considered positive. This procedure is designed to reduce
   the likelihood of a false positive test result.
4. If the initial test is finally determined to be positive (as
   defined above), the Western blot test is performed.
5. If the Western blot test is negative, the patient is advised that
   the initial test result was most likely a false positive and that
   there is no *evidence* of infection at the current time.
6. If the Western blot is positive, the patient is informed that
   there *is* evidence of HIV infection.

An important source of inaccurate test results has to do with the
biology of the disease rather than with the limitations of laboratory
testing. This is the time lag between infection and development of
detectable antibodies (by *any* test). Most infected people (more than
95%) will develop detectable antibodies within six months of infection. However, there are some persons who don't develop detectable

antibodies until even later. During the time between infection and development of antibodies, the disease can still be transmitted to others (by the routes described in the transmission section of this chapter). Unfortunately, both initial and confirmatory tests during this time yield negative results. These are called *false negative* test results.

False negative test results are most often a problem in persons who have *recently* engaged in high risk behavior (for example, sharing of dirty intravenous needles, practice of receptive anal intercourse) that could have resulted in infection without enough time to have developed detectable antibodies by either test. Therefore, if there has been recent "high risk" behavior by a person who tests negatively for HIV, retesting in three to six months is often recommended. Repeat testing is not usually recommended for persons with negative results from both tests and no evidence of "high risk" behavior. These persons should be counseled about "high risk" behavior and advised to avoid such.

False *positive* test results are primarily a problem in persons at "low risk" for infection (for example, those who confine sexual practice to a monogamous relationship). These persons usually give true negative results by the confirmatory Western blot. However, there are some conditions which can cause difficulty in interpreting the Western blot test, such as other retroviral infections, autoimmune diseases, chronic inflammation that results in production of excessive antibodies, presence of antibodies that react with white blood cells, and certain types of liver disease.

All persons who test positively by the initial test and by the confirmatory test should be referred to a doctor specializing in infectious disease and skilled in the care of HIV-infected persons. It is also important to choose a doctor who understands the limitations of testing and the causes of false test results.

Testing for HIV infection will continue to improve with greater elimination of false test results. The major direction of improvement will be toward developing tests that directly detect the virus, or parts of the virus, rather than depend on indirect evidence of infection (the antibody response).

Finally, it is important to remember that the quality of any test result depends on the quality of the laboratory performing the test. There are a number of laboratory certifying agencies, sponsored by both the government and professional societies, that serve to assure quality lab results. However, if you have any concern about the reliability of your test result, ask you doctor to find out if the laboratory performing the test is regularly inspected and properly certified to do highly accurate HIV serologic testing. There are rigorous quality assurance programs for laboratories that do HIV testing, and inspections are designed specifically to determine the accuracy of a laboratory's HIV test results.

Do whatever you need to do to allay your doubts and uncertainties about the accuracy of your HIV test result. Don't ever be afraid or embarrassed to ask for a repeat test if you feel a mistake has been made. Too much is at stake to accept such important news blindly. Discuss your doubts and concerns immediately with your personal physician.

Chapter 3

Facing and Sharing
Test Results and Diagnosis

Soon after receiving a confirmed "positive" HIV test result or diagnosis of AIDS, you will probably ask yourself, "Should I tell anyone about this?" There will certainly be those you should not tell. A family member, friend, or coworker might be too old, too young, or too emotionally fragile to accept the news. Others should and will need to be told as soon as you are able, whatever your reservations about their reactions.

People are suprisingly resilient. Most find ways to deal with the realities of illness and the possibility of death, even when it involves those they love most. They find the inner strength to face seemingly unbearable grief. The first person to consider, however, is yourself. You must face your own reality, find your own inner resources, and develop your own coping skills. The time will come when you can include loved ones and friends, who can then assist you in developing an expanded support group.

The news that you actually have HIV infection, or AIDS, hits everyone with waves of shock, panic, and disbelief. But each person needs a different amount of time to pull thoughts together and to deal with the reality of AIDS. In reading the sections that follow, you should remember that only you really know your emotional time-table. Think about sharing as soon as you are ready to do so.

A Time to Talk and a Time for Secrets

Confidentiality has been a primary concern since the first few cases of AIDS were diagnosed. With the scientific assurance that transmission of HIV was limited, and preventable, came greater understanding and acceptance of those who were infected, but fear and prejudice remain in every community, and will probably be found within your own circle of acquaintances, co-workers, and friends. Often the worst breaches of confidentiality occur not because of carelessness on the part of clinics, physicians, or insurance companies, but because patients themselves have confided in the wrong people. Choose your confidants wisely. Be careful that in reaching out for the support you need, you don't create additional problems for yourself.

Landlords have asked persons with AIDS to vacate their apartments, public utility companies have refused them services, and community leaders have even at times branded them threats to the public welfare. Always ask yourself, "Do *I* have a need for this person to know?" before you ask, "Does *this* person have a need to know?" Consider your own security first, and then the needs of the other person.

When Should You Share the News?

On a practical level, trying to hide the diagnosis from those close to you is usually fruitless. As you move from hope to despair, and back again, family and close friends will sense something is deeply troubling you, even before they learn the facts.

Most people with AIDS have found the best choice is to share the diagnosis and to give those closest to them the opportunity to offer their support. They have found it easier, in the long run, to express their fears and hopes, than to try to hide them. In telling the people you love that you are HIV-positive, or have AIDS, you give them the opportunity to express their feelings, and to extend a helping hand. Of course, you must use words and timing that you find comfortable to tell others what you are going through. Try to share your news with them as soon as you feel ready. Choose a close friend in whom you can safely confide, and ask for help in talking with others.

There are undoubtedly family members, friends, and coworkers who should *not* know, or who have no need to know the specific details of your medical or personal situation. Your needs must be considered first for your own well-being and peace of mind.

If you have no family, it is especially true that the road appears less lonely when shared with a few close friends. You might lose one or two: some people will find it too difficult to talk with you or be around you, and they will slip away. On the other hand, you may discover hidden strengths and compassion in the least likely of companions.

One man with AIDS wrote, "I think you learn quickly whom you can talk to. Some people make themselves scarce if AIDS is mentioned. But, people with AIDS soon learn who their trusted friends are."

A father of three young boys told me, "When I was diagnosed with AIDS I could not talk to them about it. It was just, well, the idea of maybe not being here to see them have their own children, and be a grandpa, and see them get married, and get through college or whatever they were going to do with their own lives, was really traumatic, because I had so much wanted children, and I wanted to be the best dad in the world. I felt after I confronted my wife with my gayness that from that point on I could face almost anyone. I didn't realize how difficult it was going to be until I faced the issue of not only being gay, but having AIDS, with my three children. And so it took me a couple of months before I was really able to even think about telling them. And through therapy and through dealing with this issue I realized the only way I was going to have complete peace was in fact to discuss it with them."

Another young man remarked, "We're all learning to communicate. In fact, this disease is making the whole world communicate.

We think we communicate all our lives but we don't. We don't want to hurt somebody's feelings . . . so we don't say anything at all. And my whole family's learning. We didn't cry with each other for a year! We were all being strong for each other and you've got to get that out because all it does is manifest inside." Yet another added, "I don't think you should keep it to yourself. I wasn't the only one who needed to talk. My family and friends needed to share their feelings and were afraid to ask me if we could talk about it. Life is very short for everyone, at best. Since there are no guarantees, we should make the most of each day."

When the Family Finds Out First

On rare occasions, when critical illness strikes a patient who didn't know he was infected, family members may be the first to learn the diagnosis. If, as a family member, you are the one to decide, should you tell the patient? Some might think not, but most people with AIDS disagree. "I don't care how sick the guy is, I think anyone with AIDS should be told the truth," one patient wrote. "Time is so valuable, and there may be things the person would like to accomplish. There are decisions to be made. . . ."

All of us have important life choices to make. People with AIDS sometimes find these choices become crystal clear when they feel their life span could be cut short, but others need time to re-evaluate goals and plans for the future. Although such patients may outlive any one of us, people with AIDS have the right to know, and to decide how they will spend their remaining days. Naturally, there are exceptions to any generalization, but most people relate that "Ted took the news much better than we thought he would."

A man who himself has AIDS recalled how public attitudes and perceptions have changed, even in the relatively short time since his critically ill roommate was diagnosed with AIDS in 1984. "It's true that Stephen was very very sick, but his relatives never told him that they knew he had AIDS. They didn't get uptight about him being gay, but even among themselves they kept calling this disease a rare form of leukemia. And they kept saying he would get better. Of course, then, they didn't have the treatment for opportunistic infections they have available now. Looking back I realize that he should have tried to open up too. But by not telling him that they knew, everyone was deprived of a chance to work things out. A lot of opportunities were lost."

Family members also bear great emotional burdens after learning the diagnosis. They, too, need the comfort of sharing their feelings. Yet, it is almost impossible to support the rest of the family if you are hiding the diagnosis from the person with AIDS. And he or she inevitably learns the truth. Often they suspect the possibility of AIDS even before they show any signs of illness. The consequences of secrecy can be deep anger, hurt, or bitterness. The patient may believe that no one is being honest because "AIDS is always terminal." And, while you are trying to save the patient from anxiety, the patient may be trying to protect family and friends from learning the truth. Then everyone ends up suffering alone, with thoughts and feelings locked inside.

Mutual Support and Responsibility

Clearly, the most compelling reason for sharing the diagnosis of AIDS with your friends and family is that AIDS can be so terribly lonely. No one needs to try to bear it alone. Yet you may feel that your illness is an exception. Perhaps you fear that prejudiced or ignorant individuals will seek to attack you, or to pass moral judgment on your worth as a human being. It is true that there will be times when you will feel totally without friends or comfort, regardless of the number of people offering you support, but there is no need to make things harder by putting on a facade meant to convince others close to you that you do not need their help.

You must not shut people out when they are trying to cope with your illness, and when they also need your support. Talking about your needs, and asking questions of others, builds a foundation of mutual understanding to sustain you through the struggle ahead.

You can, and should, share anxiety and sorrow, but you can also share love and joy, and express your appreciation for each other in ways you ordinarily might overlook or find difficult or embarrassing. By sharing and listening, you will be more aware when others need your support and reassurance.

Friends create a vital support team to protect you from the cruelty of the thoughtless, help you work through problems when you feel uncertain and confused, and back up your decisions when others doubt you.

One young man, hospitalized for weeks, was growing more and more angry with the continuous stream of people passing through his room. Hospital students, distant relatives not seen in years, and friends who thoughtlessly brought *their* friends by to visit were draining his strength and taking away precious time on the days he did feel able to do things for himself. Only after he explained in tears that he wanted a little less "attention" did his family begin to help protect him, as well as support his needs.

Your close companions can't be expected to be mind readers, but they want to help. Only when you are honest with your feelings, and are willing to share your frustrations, can you expect effective support.

Chapter 4

The Multiple Issues of AIDS

Learning that your physical condition has changed because of a life-threatening viral infection (HIV) may forever alter the things you believed in the past. It is an end to the innocence you may have projected into the future, especially if your infection is the totally unexpected result of a contaminated blood transfusion. But it can also be a beginning. A renewed evaluation of goals, and an enriched perspective of the value of the future is not only possible, but essential to your mental well-being.

If there seem to be too many problems confronting you all at once, this is the moment to begin sorting them out and setting priorities. Make lists of questions to resolve for yourself first, and then take your feelings and decisions into an extended family discussion, or to your physician or therapist, for review and guidance. A mountain of multiple concerns may look like an impossible obstacle. However, viewed separately, each problem will be more easily solved. In any case, set your own time schedule, and work with only as much as you can handle at this moment.

There are no better examples than real-life situations encountered and faced by others. The more specific discussion of the many issues of AIDS that follows includes personal feelings shared by patients and their families as they lived through those first weeks of anxiety following a positive HIV test result.

In the Beginning

This isn't possible! There has been a mixup of test results! I said that over and over to myself. I wasn't gay, I didn't use drugs. My transfusion was in a small town hospital. Something was wrong! I went for almost six months without telling anyone or mentioning my feelings to even my doctor. I stopped seeing my friends, didn't spend Christmas with my family, and almost lost my job. I didn't want to do anything but sleep. Then I met this other guy with a test result like mine. I had wasted so much good time. I never knew so many people would be so helpful. If only I had been brave enough to ask questions.

There is increasing evidence that repeat testing may be worthwhile. Monitoring the immune system is extremely important so that early diagnosis and treatment for opportunistic infection is possible. But if you have doubts about your test, go immediately to your doctor. Ask questions. Repeat the test if it will give you peace of mind. Then, if positive test results are confirmed, begin the process of building a support group as soon as possible. You should never try to face the many uncertainties of AIDS alone.

"Have I infected everyone I've had sex with?" I asked myself that question a million times. The fear and guilt I felt over possibly infecting past sexual partners made it impossible for me to even leave the house. I knew I had to talk to a few of them, but I couldn't live with the idea that they would hate me . . . I just knew someone would blame me for purposely going out and hurting people. Thank God, I found a counselor who understood and helped me. I almost committed suicide over something that never happened.

If fear for the welfare of others can't be handled alone there are many agencies and professionals prepared to help out in just such situations. In many cases, public health groups can help notify individuals with the news that they may have been exposed, without revealing your identity. Ethical issues are very real. Others who may have been unintentionally exposed have a right to know as quickly as possible so that they too may prepare for the necessary lifestyle changes and medical care. We all bear a responsibility for slowing the spread of this disease, and for seeking professional help when the going gets too tough.

"I don't need a counselor. I handle things just fine by myself!" Boy was that a cop-out. I had to get really sick twice and lose fifty pounds before I finally said, "I can't make it by myself." I guess I always thought a therapist was there to take away the control over my own life. I didn't know how good she would be at helping me see that it was the feelings and fantasies about things that weren't real that needed control.

. . .

I knew I deserved to be punished, but why did God let this happen to me? I never really said that to anybody out loud. I just assumed that I was being punished for past sins! I just kept saying I was sorry for all the bad I'd done, but the problems didn't go away. Then a nurse at the hospital asked me why I thought I was so important. She wanted to know why a baby downstairs was dying, and what the baby had done. I really was mad that she was so rude. But really, she was so right! For me, it was understanding that there was a real important reason for accepting responsibility for what I did that exposed me to a virus instead of constantly dwelling on the thought that I was so much worse than the rest of the world that I didn't deserve to live.

. . .

Nothing is ever going to be the same! Of course that is true, you know. Everything is different. But at the time I was so scared of that word "nothing," that I didn't even take a minute to figure out what had really changed. It turns out lots of things that are really good, important parts of my life haven't changed at all! But one thing—I make time count a lot more than I ever did before. And that's a change I kind of like!

For some, the changes are dramatic and sudden. A successful business executive shared with us:

> I was tested on a Monday. On Tuesday, I found out the results; that I was, in fact, positive; that they were going to run a confirmatory test, the Western Blot. It came back on Thursday and on Friday I was in the hospital with Pneumocystis and nearly passed away the following Wednesday. So, it was fairly dramatic. In fact, it was the most impacting time to this point in my life. It absolutely changed everything about my entire life. It created a great deal of fear in everyone involved; a lot of heartache. But the positive side of it is that I learned, with good therapy, that you can deal with anything—even death, staring you in the face.

. . .

> I'll lose my job, insurance, friends, family! I was sure it was all over. Of course, I did lose some things; a few people left right away. At one point I had to fight for my insurance to cover one bill I had. But the PWA Coalition helped a lot with the important stuff. I only get real uptight when I try to handle it alone. Sometimes you have to look for help, but I've never had to look for very long. There's a lot of people who care.

. . .

> "Oh well, at least now I know I can't get AIDS from anybody—I've got it!" Back when I said that to myself, I hadn't even stopped to think about exposing somebody else. I knew I was HIV-positive and so I figured I'd just be careful. I was lucky. Somebody explained that I did not have AIDS. I'd been infected, sure. But taking chances could expose me to additional infections, other venereal diseases. I admit, I was pretty slow about starting to think about others or even what my test meant. Now I talk about it every chance I get. Complacent attitudes are deadly. People have to know how important this is. I pray I don't ever get really sick, but I know I'd feel a lot better if I just keep one other person from being infected. I get really political about it now. I even make enemies. That's okay.

I really feel good about the work I'm doing, and when I feel like it, I talk about it. No more holding it in and saying it doesn't exist!

Addiction

If you are using illegal drugs, or feel that you may be involved at any stage of drug addiction, get help now! HIV infection need not be a death sentence, but foreign chemical substances in the bloodstream will defeat your immune system, and combined with HIV infection, you are certain to develop medical complications if you don't attend to your health immediately.

Perhaps you've admitted to yourself that you always knew the drugs would catch up with you somehow, but not in this way. The rising panic you feel is normal and natural, but it is not something you can afford to ignore. Seek out professionals who understand your addiction and can give you the facts about your infection. Learn what HIV infection and AIDS really mean! You will not be the first person who has faced and conquered addiction; you can restore your health and purpose for living.

Addiction coupled with HIV infection presents one of the most complicated problems a family member or concerned friend can face when trying to understand or provide assistance. Keep in mind that HIV infection comes about as a result of sharing needles. It is not the use of drugs that exposes the body to this infection but the exchange of body fluids—in this case, blood. We are, however, discussing the multiple issues of AIDS, and this virus knows no difference between healthy well-adjusted individuals, and persons suffering from any number of addictive substances, whether alcohol, pills, or intravenous drugs.

In most cases, your approach to the drug user must be more confrontational because he is constantly anesthetized, and his denial system, reinforced by drugs, might as well be made of concrete. Whether the drug of choice is cocaine, crack, or speed, the addict is not well oriented to his environment, denial of reality has become an integral part of his personality, and his attention span is much shorter than normal. Violent aggression is not uncommon. Use of other substances, such as heroin, may be less disruptive to observable behavior patterns, but the heroin user's somewhat more organized approach adds the potential complication of illegal activities such as theft or assault in order to obtain the needed drugs.

The addict will jump to radical assumptions of what HIV infection or a diagnosis of AIDS means. Addicts' fantasies about the unknown will be far worse than reality. Because such individuals suffer from self-destructive personality disorders, they will be inclined to compound their already complex problems in ways that will insure failure.

The addict faced with crisis will most likely dive into his addiction. Once high, he will do everything possible to stay high—and often what appears to have been a suicide by the addict was in fact the accidental result of an attempt to find the next fix. Long binges following bad news are common, and those who have become accustomed to shooting up will use any syringe that is available.

If it seems unbelievable that anyone would avoid taking such an obvious precaution as using clean needles, keep in mind that when the fix is needed, the addict is not only in pain, but he truly believes "nothing really bad can happen to me." When addicts do consider the consequences, which is rare, they will contemplate the likelihood of being busted, having too little money for a fix, possible fights over drugs or "territory," but rarely will they consider disease as a potential enemy.

If addicts are ever willing to review the unfortunate paths of their lives, they will consider the cost of the habit in terms of dollars and cents, or energy wasted, but never in terms of opportunities or relationships lost. As one client commented about his habit, "You may think it's bad, but it could be a lot worse. I spend at max $60 a day. It could be $3,000. Besides, my wife works. We can afford it."

For the friend of IV users, there is at least some time to seek professional help. For the user of pills, time is shorter. Persons addicted to prescription drugs, or black market pills and capsules, are likely to resort to drinking as their first line of defense against reality. Because they will then follow the alcohol with pills, there is not a lot of time to provide proper suicide prevention counseling.

Alcoholics will extend their drunken binges in time of severe crisis. Those who wish to help have more time to do so, but must be aware that the alcoholic frequently has an extremely short attention span and an impaired ability to retain information. As with many other addictions, the reality that there is much that can be done may have to be repeated many times over before it sinks in.

There is much that you, as the primary supportive friend, can do. But remember that this is not the time to attack the addicted person's sense of self-worth. Labels like "drug abuser," "junkie," and the variety of derogatory street terms for alcoholics are self-defeating. Emphasizing the urgency of health care, being consistently firm and caring, just being there to provide stability can help make that vital step toward treatment possible. Don't enable the addiction—stand by the person!

Most addicts can maintain at least some kind of healthy support group; remnants of the value system learned in childhood always remain. However, that same value system that you treasure may be the very source of pain that the addict wants to avoid. Reminders of "what could have been," "wasted talent," or "disappointed family and friends" are always counterproductive until the addict honestly wants help. The past is unchangeable, but the future is a clean slate, waiting for the author to make his mark.

Find treatment centers and get information about them for your friend. Even a search through the phone book may be too great a task for him to handle. Offer to attend a session with him. Be there to talk. As one young man who was suffering from cocaine addiction remarked after several counseling sessions:

It's difficult now for me to remember that fear of the first test coming back HIV positive and then having to run the Western blot. Back then, I was wasted, and alone, even when I called the doctor's office. Then I got the results from someone who was not my physician, because he couldn't handle me at that time, and, well, it was such an unreal, strange thing for me to grasp! I mean, I needed so much more, because I was in the middle of a major addiction and was suicidal at that point. I still have no idea what that nurse said to me.

A professional treatment program can help you put a stop to addictive behavior, but equally important, such a program can also be an immeasurable help in facing mental as well as physical health problems.

Fighting addiction takes teamwork. Not choosing the many programs available only increases the odds for failure. If your friend feels he must try to "go it alone," the necessary changes, adjustments, and decisions will not be clear, nor will the reinforcement necessary be available at the times he needs it most. One individual commented about receiving his positive HIV test results:

I wanted to do more drugs. Then I didn't know what I wanted. You know, I was really kind of confused on whether I wanted to go ahead and get help, try to find a treatment, or just run an eight-ball into my arm and let it go. I mean, I literally looked back and knew I'd screwed up somewhere along the line. And this HIV is real! And now it's affecting me! And it's going to keep affecting how I'm going to live the rest of my life. And that was too heavy to handle all at once. I couldn't even make it on my own through one day!

An IV drug user who had heard horror stories about AIDS, but had always avoided those who he felt were at risk remarked:

I had lost a couple of friends who died of AIDS. We were in many high risk groups. And I shared needles; I had shared needles with them years ago. And suddenly I started to wonder, you know, what they died of . . . How they went through what they went through. Was I to blame somehow? And you know the strange part of it all? The high for me was how close to death I could get and still make it. I got too close. Now the high is making one more day clean.

There is an additional, though controversial and as yet misunderstood, type of addiction. Here, the synthetic drug has been replaced by adrenaline, and the addiction is to sex itself. As with other types of addiction, there is good, sound treatment available, and hope for the future. If you feel that you may have problems with sexual addiction, and feel unable to seek professional help, start on the road to freedom by reading the excellent books written by Dr. Patrick Carnes, listed in the reference section of this book.

The causes for addictive behavior can be as varied as the people addicted, but the results of addiction are always the same. Addiction kills. Your approach to a friend trying to conquer addiction may be different from anyone else, but above all, love strengthens resolve. Share it without qualification.

Sexual Lifestyles

Because AIDS was first identified in this country within the homosexual community, the initial repercussions were directed at the community itself, rather than at the actual disease. As a direct result, the healthy self-esteem that had taken homosexuals generations to cultivate was seriously wounded. The concept of "Gay Pride" too often gave way to conversations about the "Gay Disease," and prejudice that had previously been based on philosophical or religious differences now was falsely supported with arguments about the danger of homosexuality to the physical well-being of the community.

The truth is, if you are gay or bisexual and have been infected with HIV, it is *not* because of your sexual preference. Once again, remember: AIDS knows no boundaries. Sexual transmission occurs because of unprotected sexual activity that allows for the exchange of body fluids. It can, and does, infect men or women who do not practice safe sex, *whatever* their sexual preference: heterosexual, bisexual, or homosexual.

However, having your sexual identity labeled "out of the mainstream" or "abnormal" is undeniably an additional source of stress for you at a time when you are least able to cope with prejudice and cruel accusations from others. You may in fact, consciously or unconsciously, be too critical of yourself as well.

There is good cause for disapproval of "one-night stands," "tricks," or "pick ups," where indiscriminate and careless sexual activity can so easily spread so many forms of disease. Having said that, noted religious thinkers have insisted that the only kind of sexual ethic possible, or even desirable in this time, or any other, will rest on free, responsible, personal decision. You have a clear right, and a moral obligation, to responsible expression of your feelings and sexual preferences. Unfortunately, such rights are in most cases not supported by law. A number of difficulties must be prepared for in advance, especially by homosexual couples.

When AIDS makes it impossible to keep "Uncle Jack in the dark," you may also find it impossible to confront sexual preference issues, let alone your physical condition. Literally hundreds of papers, books, and pamphlets have been written to help you with the task of "opening the closet door," and many of the agencies in the reference section of this book can provide sources for such materials. A professional counselor can help you establish your own guidelines in sharing information about your personal life and separate what needs to be told from personal thoughts that are truly your own. Don't be afraid to let sympathetic family members intercede for you.

If you are most comfortable with your mate having sole responsibility for your shared possessions, your health care, and the many day-to-day decisions that you cannot presently handle, carefully prepare in advance any legal contracts that will make such responsibility a certainty. Consult an attorney who is knowledgeable and sympathetic to your needs. In the event of an accident that may require surgery, it can be vital that you have made provision for someone to sign for your health care needs. In the event that you are single and without family, such precautions are especially important; granting power of attorney in the event of emergency can save your life!

If you feel you may have been the victim of discrimination, whether on the job, in the community, or even in the hospital, don't assume that you are without recourse. Doctors, lawyers, counselors, and clergy are there to help you create better human conditions. Take advantage of their services.

For the gay or bisexual male, questions of adjusting to sexual expression that is safe and still fulfilling need special attention. Safe sex need not be boring, nor should sexual needs be set aside as unimportant. Find new ways to touch, embrace, and explore each other, mentally as well as physically. Read about massage, light the evening with candles, and share fantasies that caress the mind as well as the body.

The many questions that race through your mind are not solely your own. Others around you are facing the same uncertainties and fears. Support groups that allow for the open expression of your doubts and anxieties will also be the source of renewed hope and fresh approaches to unsolved problems. Don't be afraid to ask others how they cope. They may have the answer you need most, and by asking, you give them a sense of usefulness as well. No doubt some of the questions others ask will sound familiar.

What if I have infected my lover? The fear of having infected my lover was destroying me. What would his reaction to the news be? I knew I would probably lose him and that was so much more scary than worrying about what was going to happen to me! I was making myself sick worrying. When he finally couldn't stand my moods anymore, it just came out. I couldn't hold it in anymore. We cried together. We screamed. We fought, but we made it. It had almost destroyed me though, before I said anything. Those days were the worst of all.

One gay male couple came to a new and fulfilling understanding of personal commitment. Knowing that they are both HIV positive, they recently told me, "We never knew each minute could be so important; there's no time now for arguments. We have learned how to give each other some space." Not all relationships will be so "understanding," but much can be accomplished by knowing when it is time to seek professional assistance to strengthen the relationship, and to expand the support group.

If this is true, I'll kill him! I hated him for doing this to me. I decided he was a murderer and that he probably even knew he had infected me. Then one day a friend of his in my support group told me that Gary was practically desperate to see me.

Would I please go, or at least make a phone call. Would you believe that my best friend now is probably the guy I got this from? We still keep saying we're sorry all the time. But we have each other to talk to. I couldn't make it without that.

Above all, fill your life with activities that are healthy diversions. The tragedy of gay communities who watched as literally dozens of their friends became critically ill or died is unspeakable. Yet dwelling on such losses can only undermine your own strength. People with full-blown AIDS are living longer, and receiving better care every day. Others have survived. You can too. Celebrate your victories. Be innovative in creating memories that heal whenever you recall them.

Women and the Unexpected Risk

How could I have known so little about him? I mean, we have been married for thirty-six years. After all this time, how could I not have known that there was so much in his life that didn't include me? Does this mean he never loved me? What will I tell our friends, our family, the grandchildren?

It's hard to imagine more alarming news than that delivered to a woman at retirement age, married for most of her life, who had never worked outside her family, had no formal education from which to draw experience for a career, and who had to confront the realities of her husband's lifestyle, until then completely hidden from her but now exposed by AIDS. Increasing numbers of wives, unaware of the bisexuality of their husbands, are facing such stern realities. Such women may need the support and assistance of community members in order to survive.

The tragedy of the growing number of young married women who also face the news that their husbands are HIV positive is undeniable. Not only are there the issues of disease and fear of death to face, but there is the additional shock of behavior that may never have been apparent. An increasing number of wives of men who were infected with HIV through the use of contaminated needles also are facing the brutal reality of AIDS.

All who are involved in such situations need special care and understanding. Young wives may need help at home for a period of time, and certainly need the opportunity to talk freely about their doubts, fears, and anger, without prying questions or casual advice from those who have never faced such overwhelming disruption to their personal lives. Help is possible, but the difficulties are many, and professional counseling is an absolutely essential part of any treatment program. Many of the resource agencies that have so benefited persons with AIDS can be of help here as well, but it may be more difficult for the wife to seek, or to accept, such assistance.

When There Are Children

Children sense the truth. Some parents who tried to "spare" their children have later regretted not telling them the truth during the course of the disease. Children have an amazing capability to adjust when we help them understand a situation. However, when their normal world is turned upside down and whispered conversations go on behind closed doors, they often imagine situations that are worse than reality. Young children blame themselves and dwell on the "terrible" things they have done or said that have "caused" the upheaval in the family.

Children's ages and emotional maturity should be your guide in what and how much to disclose. It might help to realize that sharing the truth with children—reassuring them they are not responsible for what has happened to the family—is a great comfort to them. Including them among those who know reinforces their sense of belonging.

A parent with AIDS may want to tell the children outright: "I've been sick a lot lately, haven't I? I have a disease called AIDS. The doctors are going to do everything they can to make me healthy and strong. Sometimes I won't be able to spend as much time with you as I want to; it's going to be hard on all of us, but I still love you very much and you are a big help to me."

Perhaps this is too painful. A loving aunt or uncle, or a close friend of the family, might be able to explain things more comfortably: "Your daddy is ill. The doctors are doing everything they can to make him feel better, but sometimes the treatments make him feel sad or grouchy. It's nothing you children have done, but he needs your patience and understanding."

The goal in telling the children that someone in the family has AIDS is to give them opportunities to ask questions about the disease and to express their feelings about it. Of course, all of us want to shield our children from pain, but pain that they understand is easier for them to cope with than what they imagine. Some adults tell us that they still remember the feelings of rejection they suffered as children when someone in the family was critically ill, or an impending divorce broke down family communication. As children, they were aware of great disruption within the family, but were denied knowledge of the cause. They were hurt and confused by lack of attention on the one hand, and by what seemed to be unreasonable demands and expectations on the other. Their sense of self-worth was damaged when they believed that if they really were important to the family unit, more information would be shared with them.

Be careful in assuming what others are able to grasp, and what they have retained. A sensitive father, who, after discussing for some time his diagnosis with his sons, felt certain that his youngest boy was aware of the circumstances, and had a competent grasp of the potential difficulties ahead. He decided that a vacation trip together would be healing for everyone. On the second day of their travels, his young son broke down in tears as the family drove past a cemetery; he clutched his father's neck and sobbed, "You might die, Daddy." The process of sharing, discussing, and really listening, began anew.

Helping Friends with Complex Problems

However great the shock, depression, or grief, a series of planned steps needs to be followed to help anyone whose life has been touched by AIDS: those who have just received the devastating news of HIV infection or diagnosed AIDS—and those who love or care about them.

1. Watch for signs of mental shock. Reasoning with someone in such a mental state is futile. With virtually no attention span, and little ability to comprehend more than raw fear, the person under stress can best be helped by attending to the many household details he or she cannot handle, by a firm but loving touch, and by quiet, understanding companionship.

2. Seek immediate counsel. Not even the most competent mental health clinician could handle such news and the many questions that will follow. Seek out professionals who have experience in your particular area of need.

3. Locate support agencies in your immediate area that can help explain to you, and your friend, both the emergency situations that may arise for which you can begin to prepare, and the kind of help that is available.

4. Be available and dependable. For people in crisis, the world has turned upside down. Nothing seems solid or reliable. Your ability to appear calm and peaceful (even when you feel your own knees weakening) will provide a source of strength when the going gets particularly rough.

5. Whenever a couple is confronted with HIV, remember that there are three patients in crisis, not just two: husband and wife, or partners, and the relationship itself. All three need a great deal of loving care. As a friend, however good your intentions, you cannot meet the needs of all three. Do the best you can, and get additional help when your personal reserve is getting too thin.

6. Generalized fear of loss is frequently obvious, but some aftershocks of crisis take time to materialize. When the going gets rough, the sociability found in support groups may make the difference between a life of intensely good quality, and a life made shorter and more pathetic by stress and loneliness. After those first days, weeks, and even years, keep an eye open for doubts and anxieties that will recur.

Whether you have been infected with HIV, or are trying to be a supportive friend, face realistically only the problems of today, one at a time. Find ways to build inner fortitude as well as physical strength. Assaults on self-worth are sometimes monumental. Every television program, commercial, call from a friend, contact with family, and new day can be a reminder of potential loss or lack of purpose, unless you set real goals and make real plans for tomorrow. The attitude with which you approach each question in your own mind, and the healthy concern and acceptance you give yourself for unavoidable mistakes and misgivings, can set the stage for better dealing with the sorrows, and the joys, of the future.

Chapter 5

Balancing Needs, Sharing Feelings

Sometimes, the whole family will have guessed the truth well before a physician has made his diagnosis. Someone recognizes the symptoms, or the family doctor seems overly concerned. Nonetheless, hearing that word . . . AIDS . . . you are stunned as you never have been in your life. It is often impossible to take in the diagnosis immediately. You hear it, but somehow you don't believe it. This is a perfectly normal reaction. Your mind has a wonderful capacity for absorbing information only when it is ready to accept it.

Emotions Take Time

Not all of us operate on the same emotional timetable. One member of the family might feel the need to talk about AIDS before the others are able to. You should decide when you are ready to talk, and what topics you will discuss, but neither you nor your family should feel forced to talk.

When AIDS is first diagnosed, some people can absorb only the most basic information, and even that may need to be repeated. That's normal. You, and those around you, each have the right to digest information at your own pace and to decide when you are ready for more, when you are ready to talk about what you know or want to know. If someone in the family wants to talk about AIDS before you are ready, try to postpone the discussion without rejecting the person. "I appreciate your concern, but not yet. I can't talk yet," for example, suggests that the day will come when you *will* be ready to talk. Taking care of your own needs, which are great, while recognizing the fears and anxieties of those you love is not easy, but it's worth doing.

The period right after diagnosis is often a time of anger, fear, and emotional turmoil. You might need to sort out conflicting emotions before you can express them. Or, you might find yourself lashing out, wanting to find a target for anger and frustration. Often it is those closest to you who must bear the brunt of these outbursts. You don't want to hurt them, but you may be angry that they will live and you might die. Perhaps you assume that they will understand and endure your rage.

Family members have feelings too. They may lash back, expressing their own anger and hurt at your outbursts, at the possibility of losing you, at the burden of new responsibilities, or at their powerlessness to change the reality of the disease. As you express your own feelings, try to remember that others need to express theirs as well.

Avoid manipulating the feelings of others to suit your own needs. The times you feel the greatest confusion and helplessness will be the times you feel the greatest need for support. By all means, ask for help when you truly need it, but rather than "crying wolf" every time you feel panic rising, take a moment to seek inner guidance and reflection. It is never easy to fight fear. But even a short pause to take a deep breath can ease the pressure and keep you from needlessly alarming others.

People's approaches to disease differ. Sometimes their needs clash—some need to talk; some need to think things through—by themselves; and some even need to shut the whole subject out of their minds for a while.

In some families, everyone becomes overly considerate of everyone else's needs for time to adjust. Then, instead of meeting anyone's needs, family members end up avoiding one another, building walls just when they ought to be opening doors.

It is important to let the person infected with HIV, or diagnosed with AIDS, call the signals as to when it's time to talk. But as that person, you will find it helps to look for clues that the time may be right to discuss AIDS and how to live with it. Signs such as lingering over idle conversation, spending more time around you than usual, or even showing unusual nervousness might indicate that a family member or friend wants to talk but doesn't know where to begin. And when you talk, be sensitive to how the other person reacts, how he positions his body, or whether or not she makes eye contact. These clues will tell you whether your conversation is serving a purpose or driving someone you care about into hiding.

Some people cannot adjust their feelings and cannot help each other. Not all families can be open and sharing, and a crisis is a difficult time to be adjusting family patterns. Even so, family members may still need to air their feelings. Expressing what we feel is not always a cooperative venture. Hostilities buried for many years can suddenly surface as though the pain occurred only yesterday. This is the time to turn to one of the many sources outside the family for emotional support. A number of these sources are discussed in the chapter on seeking professional assistance.

The Family Will Adjust

The period following diagnosis is a difficult time of adjustment for family members. Each has to deal with individual feelings, while trying to be sensitive to the feelings of the person with AIDS. Being part of the family doesn't mean you can make other family members talk about their feelings before they are ready, but you need outlets, too. There are ways to encourage openness. Be ready to listen when others are ready to talk, and let your continued presence show your support. But remember, the person with AIDS sets the timetable.

When you decide to talk, you may find yourself the target of a good deal of anger and frustration. It is easier to tell yourself that you are not the cause of this hostility than it is to accept it. You know you should respond with patience and compassion, but sometimes you answer anger with anger. Even these exchanges, however, serve a valuable purpose if everyone learns through them to share their feelings.

The opposite of anger may be false cheer. In trying to lift the spirits of the person with AIDS, you may actually be cutting off his attempts to express his real feelings. Remember that lifting spirits doesn't mean burying the truth. Sensing despondency, some people rush in with assurances that "everything will be all right." But everything is *not* "all right." If you insist it is, you deny the reality of the patient's world. In response, he or she may withdraw, feeling deserted and left to face an uncertain world alone. Without meaning to, you've abandoned the one you hoped to help, just when your support is so important. By denying reality, you set up patterns that can be difficult to change. The HIV infection may be controlled, but the gulf between you can remain.

It is not uncommon early on for persons with AIDS to begin clarifying their feelings about death. Thoughts of suicide are almost universal. It is inappropriate to blame yourself for contemplating an end to your life, or for thinking, as a result, that you are somehow less resilient than others who seem to be overcoming their fear. It is equally inappropriate for friends to feel that they must prevent you from having such thoughts. Suicidal depression is normal at this early stage. The sooner it is talked about freely and openly, the sooner you can begin to think about renewing and enriching your life as an alternative to taking it.

It may help the one with AIDS to know that you share the same fears and anxieties about the uncertainty of the future. People who honestly share their feelings about the future find that once they expose them to the light, they can better accept them, and turn their energies more fully to living in the present. This is a very difficult period, but if you can share the difficulties, you will find there are more good days to enjoy together. And you are less likely to be devastated by the truly difficult ones.

Hope That Is Real

Despondency or despair will make it difficult at times to be honest with yourself about hope that is realistic. Above all, remember that you are an individual. There is a common tendency to get caught up in statistics and generalizations ("If John was so sick, I will be too"), but no two HIV infections ever develop in exactly the same way. Each individual has a different genetic makeup, immune system response, will to live, and urge to fight. These cannot be measured on charts and graphs. No one can offer any of us "forever," but there are good prognoses; with an ever-growing number of AIDS research facilities, the outlook is hopeful for better and longer lives.

You can find encouragement in promising test results and in treatments that have helped others. You can make subtle but effective changes in diet, exercise, and rest time to build and strengthen your immune system. You can make new friends, spend time with others who need your help, and begin projects that divert your mind and fulfill your need to express creative energy.

Even if the future is guarded, there will be good days, comfortable nights, and wonderful shared experiences that are real beyond any numbers. Enjoying those experiences and their memories is what living is about, not counting the number of your days.

Even when there is no obvious cause for immediate hope, you as a family member or concerned friend can still provide reassurance of continuing love and comfort. At times, "I'm here" may be the two most supportive words you can say.

Opening Up

There are different ways you can be important as a family member or friend. You can listen to expressions of feelings, or act as a sounding board for a discussion of future plans. You can help focus anger or anxiety, or help explore specific areas of concern—drug reactions, the job situation, finances, and so forth. You can be what is most needed—someone to listen and react to the patient's out-pourings, without necessarily "doing" anything. It is a difficult role, but it can be immensely rewarding.

There is another, more passive, but equally difficult role. Some AIDS patients view theirs as a private battle to be fought alone, with only their physicians as allies, and they prefer to fight their emotional battles alone, as well. But they need family and friends for silent support, as respite, shelter, or an island of normalcy. It can be draining to provide "safe harbor" from a day in the clinic or nights of sleepless panic. It can be a struggle to be forced to plan an evening out, to ask friends in, or simply to stand by in silent support. However, there may be times when this is what is needed most.

Many people think they don't know "how to act" with people with AIDS. The best you can offer is to be natural, to be yourself. Let your intuition guide you. Do what you do comfortably; don't try to be someone you are not. This in itself is comforting. Dealing with AIDS is hard enough for the patient without asking him to adapt to a new you.

The person you are, whether patient or supportive friend, has not changed. Your values are as they always were. Your sensitivities, though perhaps temporarily numbed by immediate stress, will revive. Those who know and love you will recognize you as they always have, with compassion, concern, and fond memories of the experiences you have shared.

Chapter 6

Family Adjustments

Although the disease we call AIDS has "come out of the closet," much of what we read in newspapers and magazines continues to be only about the virus itself—its probable origin, the hope for a vaccine, and new methods of treatment. Prejudice about the disease, the patients, and their lifestyles, still makes discussion of personal cases difficult. Emotional concerns are still hidden from view. Families fearing harsh treatment from friends and community members still rarely speak of their needs, or ask for help.

There has been progress since the days when children with AIDS were expelled from school and their homes were burned to force them to move, but there is still little guidance about how families can deal with AIDS on a day-to-day basis. This gap reinforces the feeling families coping with AIDS have: that they are isolated from the rest of the world. Everyone else is managing nicely while they flounder with their emotions, hide from their spouses or lovers, or find themselves incapable of relating to their children.

AIDS is a blow to every family it touches. How your family handles AIDS is determined to a great extent by how it functioned as a unit in the past. Families that are used to sharing their feelings with each other are usually able to talk about the disease and the changes it brings. Families in which each member solves problems alone, or in which one person has played a major mediating role, may have more difficulty coping.

As mentioned in the previous chapter, there are far more considerations than the disease itself, and the added stress of serious illness can raise issues, long ignored, that you may have felt were no longer important. Although you are likely to need the most support, you must also be prepared to resolve each issue, sometimes alone, but always at your own speed.

Problems within the family can be the most difficult to handle simply because you cannot "go home" to escape them. Some family members may deny the reality of AIDS or refuse even to discuss it. It is understandable that you feel deserted or unable to discuss AIDS openly.

"My brother-in-law is suffering from AIDS," one man confided. "The entire situation is depressing, and I have decided to stay away. I have not visited him. There's nothing I could offer anyway. It's bad enough that my sister and the kids have to visit him."

One man with AIDS found none of his family could help him. "My mom survived dad's heart surgery years ago, and even his death last year pretty well, but now I have AIDS, and she doesn't know how to act. Phone calls and letters expressing sympathy are not what I need. I've tried since last November to express my thoughts to my brother, but he shuts out what I am saying. I know that he's angry, about a lot of things, but I can't seem to get through to him. I've learned that's a common reaction, but it doesn't help me. He won't even let my nephew visit me."

Private counseling and AIDS patient advocacy groups, or coalitions, can provide needed support and reinforcement for you in such situations. You will learn that others have faced the same problems, and are happy to discuss their solutions with you. Most important, these resources provide an outlet for the frustrations you are facing within your family or close circle of friends.

Such groups are also available for your family and friends. Sharing a copy of this handbook is a start. Once you feel better prepared to discuss the reality of your situation, invite your loved ones to join you at a meeting, go with you to a doctor's appointment, or see your therapist or case worker.

Changing Roles

Families may have trouble adjusting to the role changes that are sometimes necessary. One woman found it overwhelming to come home from work, prepare dinner, oversee the children's homework, change bedding and dressings, and still try to provide companionship and emotional support for her children and critically ill husband.

In addition to her roles as wife, mother, and nurse, a woman might have to add a job outside the home for the first time. A spouse or lover, who previously did not need to work or provide financial assistance, sometimes becomes the sole wage earner and homemaker. The partner who was head of the household might now be its most dependent member.

These changes can cause great upheavals in the ways family members interact. The sheer weight of responsibility can become unbearable, crushing normal family associations, devouring time needed for rest and recreation, and depriving family members of constructive expression of anxiety and resentment. The usual patterns are gone.

Parents may look to children for emotional support at a time when the children themselves need it most. Teenagers may have to take over major household responsibilities. Young children can revert to infantile behavior as a way of dealing with the impact of AIDS.

Watching for Signs

Breakdown of the family unit varies in intensity from one family to the next, but warning signs are usually obvious early on. If you have no immediate blood relatives and have "adopted a family of friends," communication problems can be just as real. For everyone involved in the family unit there are signs to watch for:

1. Has the normal pattern of daily activity changed substantially? Are family members still sharing meals together? Are there more frequent times when each person retreats into privacy? Are some members of the family spending too many evenings outside of the home?
2. Is communication difficult? Is there less open conversation than there used to be? Has everyone stopped asking sensitive questions?
3. Are arguments more frequent, and are they based on unimportant issues? Are such disagreements resolved, or set aside?
4. Is there an organized approach to household duties, or are responsibilities just assumed?

Performing too many roles at once can endanger emotional wellbeing and the ability to cope. Select problems that need immediate attention first. Make changes in routine and responsibility that will allow for more productive use of your time. For example, you can relax housekeeping standards, or learn to prepare simpler meals. Perhaps, if you have a family, the children can take on a few more household chores than they have in the past.

If a simple solution is not enough, consider getting outside help for practical assistance as well as for setting priorities and encouraging the participation of all family members. Licensed practical nurses can help with the patient; county or private agencies can provide trained homemakers. If outreach is an important part of your church, feel free to ask for help with cooking, shopping, transportation, and other homemaking tasks. One young man in poor health was adopted by his church youth group when they learned of the extra difficulties he was experiencing. Everyone benefited from the relationship.

Don't assume that everyone is too busy, or preoccupied, or unable to rise to the task at hand. Generalities born of stress can prevent you from asking for help when you need it the most.

Let someone who can be objective help you sort out necessary tasks from those that can go undone. Hiring a service to help out may seem to be an unnecessary additional expense to you. After all, you've always cooked meals, washed the laundry, and run the errands yourself, and it didn't cost anything. In times of stress, however, the financial cost of help, including professional services such as counseling and nursing care, may need to be weighed against the emotional and physical cost of shouldering the load alone. It is important to remember that the family is still a unit. If the family's strength is sapped, the patient suffers, too.

Family Rights

The San Diego chapter of Make Today Count, a mutual support group for patients and families, compiled many years ago a "Bill of Rights for the Friends and Relatives of Cancer Patients," which applies equally well today for those who care for persons with AIDS. From their example, we propose the following guidelines for dealing with family burdens:

1. When caring for an AIDS patient, you have the right and obligation to take care of your own needs. Even though you may be accused of being selfish, you must do whatever you can to keep your own peace of mind. In doing so, you can better care for the needs of the patient. Each family member or friend will have different needs. These needs must be satisfied. The patient will benefit, too, by having a more cheerful person to take care of him.

2. You, as relatives and friends, have the right to determine, for yourselves, the limits of your strength and endurance, and to obtain assistance from outsiders, even if the patient objects.

3. You have the right to a life of your own. When you know that you are already doing all that can reasonably be expected of you in caring for the patient, you can have a clear

conscience in maintaining contacts with the rest of the
world.

4. If the patient attempts to use his illness as a weapon, you
   have the right to reject that behavior and do only what can
   reasonably be expected of you.

5. You have the right to set priorities for the things that need
   doing immediately. If you respond only to the geniune needs
   of the moment—both your own and those of the patient—
   the stress associated with the illness can be kept to a minimum.

Children Have Special Needs

Children have special difficulty coping with an AIDS patient. It
might be a friend at school, which could be as difficult to understand
as illness in the home. A brother they depended on for support might
be gone from the house—in a hospital that may be hundreds of miles
from home—or home in bed, in obvious discomfort, and perhaps
visibly altered in appearance. Issues of prejudice might arise that
children can't comprehend on their own.

In the face of this upheaval, children are often asked also to
behave exceptionally well: to "play quietly," to perform extra tasks,
or to be understanding of others' moods beyond the maturity of their
years. Some may resent the loss of attention. Some fear the loss of
their parent, brother, or friend, and begin to imagine their own
death. Some children, formerly independent, may become anxious
about leaving home and parents. Discipline problems can arise as
children attempt to command the attention they feel they are missing.

It may help if a favorite relative or family friend can devote extra
time and attention to the children, who need comfort, reassurance,
affection, guidance, and discipline. Trips to the zoo are important,
but so is regular help with homework and someone to attend the
school play. Young people tend to see misfortune as divine punish-

ment for their own failures; they will need concerned loved ones to help them understand what is happening, and why.

If your efforts to provide support and assurance fail, professional counseling for a child, or for child and parent together, may be necessary and should not be overlooked.

Chapter 7

Accepting Guidance When You Need Help

Which one of us did not feel that the world stopped turning when AIDS struck us? But somehow life goes on. During the period of active treatment a pressing number of decisions need to be made, questions must be answered and arrangements handled.

There are medical questions. There might be confusion or disagreement over the diagnosis. What did the doctor really mean to say? What do various terms mean? What is the outlook for remission or recovery?

It is vital, if you have been infected with HIV, that you continue to study methods of treatment. Remember, *a positive HIV test result is not an imminent death sentence!* In the spring of 1988, Dr. Bernard Bihari, director of the Kings County Addictive Disease Hospital in New York, stated, "Probably 80% to 85% of asymptomatic seropositives who use treatments can prevent symptoms from occurring. In the next two to four years, we will have interventions to stabilize people and heal their impaired immune systems. I feel very optimistic." You can, and should, share such optimism, for your own mental well-being, and as encouragement to those who suffer with you in facing the unknown. Hope heals.

Financial burdens can be crushing. Transportation to and from treatment can be a major, frustrating obstacle. Who will shop for groceries, pick up the mail, contact friends, take care of the yard? Where do you get a hospital bed, a night nurse, a person to look after the children?

The stress of handling such responsibilities can be enormous. A new kind of communication and acceptance becomes necessary. Asking for and accepting outside help may be an entirely new role for some. "Going it alone" is seldom the only recourse. If you feel that asking for help makes you appear to have lost control, remember that maturity and strength come from deciding which chores you can handle on your own, and which can be delegated to others.

You may not know whom to turn to. You may feel uncomfortable asking for help—even from agencies that were designed precisely for situations such as you now face. So where *do* you turn?

Asking Questions and Seeking Treatment

Physicians or nurses are good sources of answers to medical questions. If you have asked once and are still uncertain, ask again. If you need to, get a second opinion. The list of agencies and advocacy groups at the end of this handbook can provide additional medical resources, as well as proper channels to obtain answers to legal questions.

It's helpful to write down on a sheet of paper all the questions you have about AIDS, its treatment, possible side effects and any limitations treatments might place on your activities. (Incidentally, there may be surprisingly few limitations other than those caused by changes in physical capability or endurance.) Other members of your treatment team—counselors, physical therapists, nutritionists, radiation technologists and such—can explain the whys of their particular therapies.

Writing questions down makes them easier to remember at the next doctor's appointment. It's also helpful to call the office beforehand to alert the receptionist that you will need extra time for your appointment. This will allow you to ask all the questions you need to, and to hear all the answers. Make sure you can remember what is said. Some people take notes, some use a tape recorder, some bring along a clear-thinking friend or relative. The point is to depend on something more reliable than your own memory at a time when emotions are likely to overwhelm you.

Fear of being considered ignorant or pushy has kept many people from asking their doctor about a most important topic—the unorthodox treatments they read about in magazines or hear about from friends. You may be urged by well-meaning people to try methods that will spare you any pain or discomfort. Yet they never seem to be available through your personal physician. If you are being pressured to abandon the care you are now getting, but haven't discussed it with your doctor because you think it will insult "establishment medicine," you might try this approach: "I keep hearing about the herbal tea treatment for AIDS. Can you tell me why it isn't accepted by most American doctors? Why do some people think it works, and others believe it won't? What are the possible side effects?"

What you have asked for is information. You haven't attacked the treatment you are getting now, nor the professionals who are treating you. And if you are comfortable with the answers you get, it will help you respond when others urge you to try these methods.

Research produces treatments that are eventually proven to be without merit, as well as those that heal and promote better health. Any ailment included in the list of "incurable" diseases draws a great deal of attention from the medical and scientific community and becomes the focus for experimental treatment. AIDS is only one of the many disease conditions thus categorized, including such common diseases as arthritis, Alzheimer's disease, systematic lupus, multiple sclerosis, cerebral palsy, cystic fibrosis, and numerous forms of cancer; all attract special research and innovative treatment programs. This is not meant to deny the gravity of AIDS and HIV-related illnesses, but only to point out that searching for new and effective "answers" is not unique to this illness. Therefore, you should thoroughly investigate any experimental program before volunteering to be a part of it. If you, a friend, or a family member has an HIV-related illness, and are contemplating experimental treatment, there are a few common sense guidelines (as proposed by the American Foundation for AIDS Research) that should be kept in mind:

1. Beware of extravagant claims or promises of miraculous results. When and if a drug, agent, or technique is developed that produces proven results, it will not remain a secret for very long.

2. If an experimental treatment or therapy is offered to you for a price, be cautious. Except in special circumstances, federal law prohibits the sale of experimental drugs or agents. While a drug is being tested, the manufacturer or developer is generally obligated to produce and supply it to trial centers free of charge. In drug trials, most drug manufacturers or trial sponsors agree to pay for all testing and medical monitoring that is required. When testing would have been required even *without* the experimental treatment, the patient may be charged for certain limited costs. Ethical practitioners do not seek to profit from a treatment that is experimental. If you are requested to pay extravagant fees or "expenses" to be enrolled in a treatment program, you should consider carefully before agreeing.

3. If "mainstream" medicine can't deliver guaranteed results, what about "alternative" techniques and therapies? Good nutrition, vitamins, meditation, or mental imaging may all play a role in healing for many individuals. It has been demonstrated that emotional depression can suppress the immune system. However, beware of extravagant claims, excessive costs, or extreme regimens. Too much of anything, even water, can hurt you.

Too many persons fail to ask the medical questions most important to their physical and emotional well-being for fear of taking up the doctor's valuable time, or looking ignorant. Some say, "I'm sure he told me all of this once before." Of course, you want to be a good or cooperative patient! But the point is—it's *your* body. It's your life. And you have every right to ask as many questions as you like, as often as you like!

A well-informed patient is better able to understand his or her therapy, the possible side effects, and any unusual signs that should be reported to the doctor. A good approach can be simply to admit that you are asking for a repeat of information: "I'm pretty sure you told me some of this before, but some things didn't make sense to me then. I was so shocked. Now, I think I'd feel better if we talked about it more."

Some are ready to hold this conversation sooner than others. Some ask a few questions at a time, absorbing each piece of information before they are ready to go on. Some never ask directly. (If so, someone in the family should speak with the doctor to learn the extent of the disease or infection and the outlook for the future.) But sooner or later, in whatever way you find comfortable, it's important to let the doctor know that you understand you are HIV positive, or have AIDS, and want to talk about it.

In an ideal world, all physicians would be patient, understanding, and able to sense your every mood. They would all be available twenty-four hours a day, seven days a week. They would know when to bring out the X-ray films and lab tests, and when to draw only the sketchiest and most attractive picture of your case. They would have an unlimited amount of time to wait until you were ready to ask questions, and then would gently help you to phrase them in just the right way.

In the real world, physicians admit that they wait for cues from you, the patient. They need you to tell them what you want to know and what problems you face. Physicians are not mind readers. Whether you like it or not, it is usually up to you to take the first steps toward open communication with your doctor.

As a matter of fact, books and courses for AIDS specialists— physicians, nurses, therapists—are beginning to emphasize the importance of recognizing the feelings of the person with AIDS. Nonetheless, each person is different, and no textbook can describe your unique needs.

When It Is Time to Change Physicians

Some physicians have never learned to speak comfortably with patients or families who are facing life-threatening illness. These physicians may appear to be abrupt, aloof, or uncaring, even when they are not.

Nonetheless, if a lack of communication creates a barrier, you might be wise to seek referral to someone else. When fighting AIDS, you have to work as part of a team. Lack of trust restricts you and your doctor. It is important, however, to let the doctor know you wish to see someone else—even to ask him or her for a referral. The physician is probably also aware that a relationship based on trust and open communication has not been established.

It is also appropriate to ask your physician to suggest other doctors for a second opinion before deciding on treatment, or as a backup for those times when your own physician will not be available.

Unfortunately, there are still doctors who believe that AIDS is inevitably fatal and that "nothing can be done." If your doctor is such a person, it is only common sense to ask for referral to an AIDS specialist or to a medical facility that has a specialized AIDS treatment program.

Family physicians with extensive experience in treating AIDS and its related diseases now believe that many of the patients who are HIV positive today will live out their lives free of further disease, and others with full-blown AIDS will live longer lives of reasonable comfort and activity. While continuing as your personal physician, your doctor will refer you to mental and physical health care specialists—pathologists, radiologists or cancer specialists—for additional treatment.

You need to be honest with yourself at those moments when you feel that adequate treatment is not being given, and accept your physician's limitations. A doctor who cannot promise complete cure is not forsaking you. And a doctor who calls in other specialists is not admitting defeat, leaving you alone, or just finding new ways to spend your insurance money. The team effort is a vital and responsible approach to professional care and treatment.

A physician who uses all available medical procedures to treat the disease, to minimize its effects, and to help you function comfortably is doing everything possible to care for your physical needs.

It can be terribly frustrating, if you seek relief from your emotional aches and pains, to be rebuffed by an otherwise excellent physician. As one man puts it, "I found it impossible to discuss the cold hard facts with my doctor. And then to make matters worse, I felt that if I told him how frightened I was, I would be considered weak or childish. It wasn't until I realized I was expecting help from the wrong person that I regained the closeness I needed with my doctor."

A decision to change physicians should be based on reality and not on a quest to find a doctor who will promise a cure and guarantee to relieve all your fears.

Just as we would not expect a physician to also be able to solve our transportation problems, we should not expect him to treat our emotional selves as well. A team effort is one in which different practitioners are included to handle different problems. No single person can be equal to all of the challenges that AIDS can pose.

Where to Find Answers

It's easier to come to grips with the reality of any crisis if we replace ignorance with information. There is much to learn about each form of the AIDS-Related Complex (ARC), about forms of treatment, about the possibilities for recovery, and about methods of strengthening the immune system. Well-prepared with the facts, you are less likely to fall prey to worthless "cures," or to depressing and sometimes biased stories of what has happened to others with AIDS. Often the more you know, the less you have to fear, and the greater your opportunity to help dispel rumors born of prejudice.

Local libraries, voluntary agencies (such as Shanti, AIDS coalitions, the American Cancer Society or the Red Cross), and major AIDS research and treatment institutions, such as the American Foundation for AIDS Research (AmFAR), can be good sources of information on AIDS and its treatment. Depending on your desire for information and your ability to understand scientific terms, you can get anything from short, concise pamphlets to scientific papers.

It's a good idea to share the fruits of your research with your own doctor. AIDS is a complex set of diseases; the treatment and subsequent side effects are likely to differ with each person.

On a national level, the National Cancer Institute (NCI), which is part of the National Institutes of Health, and the National AIDS Information Clearing House (NAIC) operate information offices for the public and can answer many general questions about AIDS, its diagnosis, and treatment. In addition, you should seek out appropriate specialized facilities close to where you live. Many will have written materials and information about local self-help and service organizations for AIDS patients and their families.

The American Foundation for AIDS Research (AmFAR) maintains a list of excellent medical facilities and health teams that are conducting research into new methods of AIDS treatment. They can suggest not only institutes, but also specialists with whom your own physician might wish to consult. However, information staff members cannot offer medical advice or arrange for referral to a specific physician or institute.

The names, addresses, and phone numbers of these and many other sources of information described in this section can be found in the appendix at the end of this handbook.

Counseling Is for Everyone

"Therapy? You have to be crazy to need therapy!" Such misconceptions abound. Counseling should provide hope, help you regain your sense of dignity, face problems honestly, and give you the means to improve the quality of your life. Counseling is not the removal of your own sense of control; rather it is needed assistance in finding the inner "tools and talents" that support your self-reliance.

If you are considering being tested for HIV infection, you need to be carefully prepared and supported in your decision. You need to know the honest facts and possible implications of the testing process *before* you're tested, and your decision must be based on the most up-to-date information available.

Counseling is most essential when the results of a blood test show HIV infection. Counseling provides you with ways of dealing with the panic, anxiety, and hostility felt by you, your family, friends, and loved ones.

Some persons engaged in high risk behavior may become infected with HIV but cannot, or will not, be tested. These people, frequently including intravenous drug users and prostitutes, need to be counseled without prejudice and in a way that will reduce the risk of their contracting the infection or passing it on to others.

Counseling is also vital if you are tested and found *not* to be infected. Such test results can sometimes lead to feelings of "permanent immunity" and to high risk behavior. Others need help dealing with the guilt and anxiety of "good health" when someone close to them may be suffering from the disease.

Obviously, AIDS counseling is not just for those who are ill. A research study conducted at St. Mary's Hospital in London has shown that HIV-infected, but otherwise healthy, persons often experience more anxiety and stress than those who have developed ARC or AIDS. Counseling is essential to motivate positive behavioral changes, to establish and review practical goals, and to help you recognize the value of your achievements.

It is reasonable to say that you will cope with AIDS as you have coped with other problems. You can come to terms with the reality of AIDS, just as others have. After the initial diagnosis or treatment, you will find you are somehow able to continue your normal working and social relationships. Or, as one psychologist put it, people with AIDS learn to get up in the morning and discover that it is possible to brush their teeth, even knowing that they have AIDS. You will find, sometimes to your amazement, that you can laugh at bad jokes, and become totally absorbed in a good movie or a football game. You can shop for a new car and celebrate receiving a promotion.

How soon you come to terms with your life, however, may depend on seeking appropriate help. Those who view professional counseling as an enabling tool, rather than as an invasion of privacy, do far better, both mentally and physically. One man commented, "I think it's absolutely imperative that a person seek out some help, and at least get through the anger stage, the hate stage, the 'why me' stage, the 'I don't care' stage. You go through different levels with this whole thing and I'm sure as life continues there will be more hurdles to climb with it, but professional help is the only way to go if you want life to be 'full of meaning,' instead of 'full of fear.' "

At times, all strength will seem to desert you. You may feel overwhelmed by this new world of uncertainties. You may find that you have lost interest in favorite hobbies or activities, viewing them as painful reminders of what will be gone if treatment is unsuccessful. You want to cope, but you need support systems beyond your own. Where do you look for such support?

It was not very long ago that emotional assistance for persons testing HIV positive was simply unavailable. Even persons with AIDS and their families discovered that mental health support was nearly impossible to find. Attention to emotional needs is a relatively recent addition to standard AIDS treatment. Now, growing numbers of hospitals routinely include a mental health professional as a member of the AIDS treatment team, or offer group counseling programs. This is a hopeful sign that says, "We have a whole person here, one with a future and a life to live. This person should be able to live as normally as possible. We must provide the emotional tools to help make that happen."

Frequently, your health care workers are experiencing many of the pressures you feel. A hospitalized veteran who was critically ill told me how cold and curt his doctor was during his brief visits. Moments later, as the patient dozed off, his doctor paused at the door and asked me for a moment of conversation. As he spoke, tears rolled down his face and he admitted, "I don't know what to say. I feel so helpless. We've done all we can, and still I lay awake nights trying to think of what I may have forgotten."

Physicians, nursing staff, health workers, friends, family, anyone who comes into social contact with HIV-infected persons or patients with AIDS, should consider the benefits of counseling and the excellent support it can provide. Counseling is now more readily available for both you and your health care team in facing the feelings of frustration and uncertainty. Clinics and hospitals recognize the awesome degree of stress that AIDS can create for you and your health care providers.

You should have no feelings of shame or hesitancy, ever, if you need to seek professional help, nor should you be surprised to find that some members of your health team are suffering with you. The team effort means sharing the frustrations as well as the victories. Medical needs should be met first, quickly and effectively. But, one function of a good counseling service is to mobilize support and refer you to service agencies and specialists that, in cooperation with your physician, will become a part of a continuing support team, a vital resource in the event that you need help to prevent loss of employment, to take advantage of educational opportunity, or to overcome social handicaps.

Several years ago, when uncertainty about the cause of AIDS was still very common, even in major hospitals, one middle-aged man commented on his first hospital visit for treatment of *Pneumocystis* pneumonia. "At first I was so sick, I didn't care what happened. But I got better, and I began to notice that nurses were avoiding me. The nurse that changed my bedding wore gloves and a mask. One orderly, or whatever he was, asked me to keep my hands away from him when he drew blood, and he even wiped off the telephone before he used it. My telephone! I had enough and exploded. I told the nurse I didn't need her attitude and the orderly to find somebody else who understood what I was going through. When a counselor finally came to visit me, he apologized for some of the staff not being better informed. But to tell you the truth, I was feeling great! I knew I wanted to live when I knew I wasn't going to let anybody treat me like a leper or an outcast again! In the days that followed, we helped each other understand."

Today many hospitals consider some form of group counseling as part of standard treatment—as necessary as an exercise class, for example. Often such programs include patient and hospital worker alike. Programs are organized in a variety of ways. Many begin within days of the diagnosis. Some groups meet only for the length of the hospital stay; others are long-term, to enable members to work through problems in the everyday world. Some are composed of people with the same complications (persons without symptom of disease, or patients, for example, with *Pneumocystis* or Kaposi's sarcoma); some are combined by type of treatment (in-hospital extended care or outpatient therapy); and some by patient age. Some are just for patients; others include spouses, family, or other loved ones.

Accept professional direction for your individual therapy program. You may be included in a group that uses music, poetry or role-playing to help you explore your feelings. Some groups will be action oriented, with "veteran" patients helping you face the same problems they once encountered. Your counseling group should be run by trained professionals so that the direction of exploration is truly helpful to each participant.

You may find it easier to explore feelings—especially those you don't want to accept, such as guilt, resentment, or intense anger—in a more private setting with a person who, without judgment, will help you understand these feelings and find ways to channel them constructively. If you want to explore your feelings in individual therapy, you will find a growing number of psychologists, psychiatrists, and psychiatric social workers specializing in counseling people affected by AIDS.

Often the problem is not an individual one. The family is a unit, and each member is affected when any one member is feeling stress. Family counseling can help absorb the shock and deal with the complexities of AIDS. It can be difficult for persons with AIDS and their family members to discuss their emotions. AIDS patients themselves have frequently identified the absence of open communication within their families as a major problem. People are particularly hesitant to express negative feelings when they fear such feelings might be interpreted as placing "fault" or "blame." None of us wants to say things that will turn out to be inappropriate. Yet the major shifts in responsibilities that AIDS brings to a family can cause great resentment by those shouldering (or incapable of shouldering) the extra burdens. Loss of accustomed responsibility or authority can also cause resentment mingled with anxiety over loss of power or self-control.

Children, especially, find that their usual roles no longer are clearly defined. Parents may not have the emotional energy to provide their usual support, love, and authority. Teenagers who are ill, and were just beginning to learn the lessons of independence, can feel torn between expressing the need to handle problems on their own and the need to remain close to a parent. Teens just discovering the wonder of love and sexual expression may suddenly find their fears of exposure to disease so monumental that they are emotionally paralyzed and cannot develop meaningful relationships. These problems become less difficult to face if the family can discuss them. Some can do this without outside help. Those who cannot should seek professional assistance, and should do so at the first opportunity.

Your physician, hospital social worker and hospital psychologist are good sources for referrals to mental health professionals in private practice who are trained to counsel individuals and families affected by AIDS. Many county health departments provide psychological services, and neighborhood or community mental health clinics are becoming common in an increasing number of cities. Community service organizations such as the United Way and the American Red Cross usually support mental health facilities. County government listings in the telephone book may include an "Information and Referral" listing, one more resource for counseling services.

Support Groups

There are numerous self-help groups, organized by people just like you, that were designed to help you overcome both the practical problems of AIDS and the feelings these problems cause. Some groups are local chapters of national organizations; others are strictly "grass roots." Some are only for patients; others include family members, lovers, and friends.

Responsible organizations working with AIDS shun a "pity" approach. They exist to help you work through your feelings and frustrations. Whether you choose to accept your situation as it is, or work to change it, you can do so within the framework of a supportive group of people who know firsthand the problems you deal with every day. They will understand, and will help you begin to take control of your own situation. Some groups offer family members an opportunity to share feelings, fears and anxieties with others bearing similar burdens. Other groups provide patients with a setting where they can express negative feelings they don't want to unload on their families.

Support groups let patients without families speak openly, release their pent-up emotions without fear of taxing existing friendships, and begin to build new and vital relationships. Some support groups provide skills, training, and helpful tips for special patients, such as those who have tumors or multiple health problems. Organizations designed primarily to offer emotional support can also provide opportunities to exchange practical information, such as how to control nausea from chemotherapy, where to purchase inexpensive clothing, or how to talk to an employer about AIDS.

A self-help group can give those recovering from ARC infections an opportunity to assist those who follow. With training, some become group counselors or discussion leaders. Many AIDS patients who have recovered from critical illnesses have found that helping others gives a needed boost to their own self-esteem. (This can be especially important after a long stretch of feeling dependent on, and at the mercy of, physicians, hospital staff, and well-intentioned but overbearing family members.)

Mutual assistance groups sometimes work with health professionals and the clergy to help them understand the special emotional needs of people with AIDS. Agencies listed in the appendix can provide the names of many mutual support or rehabilitation groups with local, as well as national, offices.

The Power of Faith

From our belief in things "unknown" we draw diverse concepts and conclusions, ranging from the painful "Why me?" to "I can fight anything." Such conscious and unconscious thoughts can leave us devastated with guilt, or empower us with great strength.

Some people find a sense of purpose in organized religion. The companionship of others with similar beliefs, and the inspirational guidance received in formal worship settings can greatly strengthen resolve. Some find new faith in a divine being, and new hope from sacred writings when AIDS enters their lives. Some find the ordeal of disease changes their faith, or that faith changes how they understand that ordeal. Others, who have never had strong religious beliefs, feel no urge to turn to religion at such a time. But all of us, in time of crisis, need support and encouragement in considering the purpose of our lives. AIDS may be your call to consider what you believe, as it was for these patients.

I never really believed much of anything. High Holy Days were great and all. Lots of food and a chance to play with my friends I hadn't seen, but I really never paid any attention unless I had to—like with my Hebrew instructor. Then this happened. You know, all of a sudden I felt like I had to believe something. I didn't even care what my parents believed, or anybody else for that matter, but I had to know what I believed! I think I could teach a class about religions of the world now. I've studied them all! And you know something, I still can't tell you a lot about rules and rights and wrongs, but I do know now I believe in God. A friend of mine used to say, "God don't make junk." Kind of dumb sounding, but God made me, and I'm doing what I'm doing for a reason, and I figure God knows that reason, even if I'm confused. Funny, I guess, but even when I feel terrible now, I know He's there. All that studying and you know what I came up with? I believe. And that's enough for me.

I'm a Christian. For as long as I can remember, I've known that God loves everybody, that He hears my prayers, and He can fill our needs. Then out of the middle of nowhere came AIDS. It shook up everything. Why weren't my prayers being answered? Why was I sick? For a while, I just decided it had all been a childish fantasy. No god would allow such suffering. Then a night nurse who liked to read to me asked if she could read some of the psalms to me one night when I was in terrible pain. You'll think this is strange, but something happened to me that night. Now, when my health is really the worst it's been, I'm not afraid anymore. There is a purpose to all of this that I think I'm beginning to understand. I have learned so much. My family is closer, to each other, and to me, than we ever were. I don't even see death as the ending I once did—I believe in rebirth. My faith in God has carried me through it all and I know I can handle anything that happens because I'm not handling it alone!

Faith in any power outside ourselves serves to motivate us to action. It opens windows to possibilities far beyond what we can achieve on our own. Whether or not you are a member of a religious congregation, you have your own values and beliefs that actually form your concept of who you are. Although that concept is sometimes expressed as "you are what you believe," there are many successful philosophers, writers, and businessmen who teach that "you *become* what you believe" as well. One patient carried his belief in personal obligations a step further:

I can't buy religion. Too much of it doesn't hold water. I think we make our own future, and that if there is anything divine, it's inside of each of us. I read The Power of Positive Thinking *a long time ago, and a lot of books like it, and they all really say the same thing: nobody gets anywhere by whining and complaining. So for right now, I give it my best, and maybe if there is some kind of life after death, I will have decided what it's going to be like even before I get there. Maybe I'm creating tomorrow today. If I am, tomorrow is going to be a lot better. I've read how other people did it. I can do it too!*

Inspirational writings have moved men and women to achieve incredible things, and, at the very least, they can lift your spirits and help you find peace of mind. Even if you don't feel the need to attend a worship service or to speak with a pastoral counselor, you should include time in your daily routine for readings that will renew your hope and sense of purpose. If books like the Bible seem too formidable, start with works by writers like Norman Vincent Peale, Dale Carnegie, Napoleon Hill, or Benjamin Franklin. Hundreds of excellent paperbacks are available that will strengthen your faith in living.

Pastoral counselors can also provide inspirational materials, and are often trained to offer practical support as well. Members of the clergy, in increasing numbers, are completing programs to help them minister more effectively to people with AIDS and to their families. Individual clergymen can provide hope and comfort, but, like physicians and lay people, they vary in their capacity to cope with life-threatening illness and the possibility of death. A religious leader untrained in AIDS counseling may, however, refer you to an associate trained to work with people with AIDS, or introduce you to another member of the congregation who can provide comfort and, perhaps, more time on a regular basis than the leader can spare.

Be honest and forthright in your search to learn from the faith of others. But understand that no single individual can answer all of your spiritual questions, any more than one person can provide for your physical and emotional needs.

The chaplain came into the room and asked right off if I had "considered the sins" that put me where I was. He told me my "lack of faith made it impossible for God to love and heal me." I'll tell you one thing, I gotta give him credit for making me so mad that I got out of bed to throw him out! I think God can probably overlook even more than I can, and I even think there's a chance He'll keep me around for a while, but no preacher is going to make up my mind or God's.

You cannot, of course, expect religious leaders to be God, or to provide divine intervention. But you can expect their honest answers to your questions, and you should accept nothing less.

Chapter 8

Changes That Start Today

The frightened man was practically pleading, "I have to have something to do, right now! I can't stand the waiting and worrying! Isn't there something I can do right this minute that will change things?" With gentle dignity, the doctor replied, "Take your feet off the sofa, and we'll talk about it."

This simple, seemingly flippant reply carries an important message. Sitting and worrying is, in itself, a decision to do nothing. It is true that nothing will seem the same from the day of diagnosis. Even if you have no signs of infection or illness, you will feel completely different. Perhaps nothing will seem real. Getting up and doing something—involving yourself in worthwhile projects—is constructive for both mind and body, and the best first step is a good plan for improving your physical health. While you are learning about treatments, you can choose good nutritional programs and exercise techniques that will improve not only your general physical health, but how you feel about yourself as well.

There are known ways you can strengthen your immune system through improved diet. Numerous books are available that identify helpful foods and nutritional supplements and their effect on the body. Some excellent ones are listed at the end of this handbook. For example, beta carotene (a vegetable precursor of Vitamin A), Vitamin C, Vitamin E, selenium, and dietary fiber are all known to be protective against cancer. From a practical viewpoint, you can start today to strengthen your immune system and improve your physical health by following these five nutritional guidelines:

1. Increase the amount of fruit, raw vegetables, and whole grain cereals in your daily diet.
2. Reduce the amount of saturated and unsaturated fat to a maximum of 30% of the total calories you consume each day. This means avoiding fried foods, butter, cream, any whole milk products, and salad dressings.
3. Avoid salt-cured or charcoal-broiled foods.
4. Remove alcohol, hydrogenated fat, refined sugar and flour, and preservatives from your diet.
5. Limit the amount of stimulants you drink, such as coffee and tea, and be conservative with hot spices. Use red pepper rather than black, which is harder on the stomach lining.

Exercise, beside building a firmer, tighter, more attractive body, is also known to strengthen the immune system. It improves circulation and speeds the elimination of toxins from your system. And don't overlook the benefits of massage as well. Not only are regular massages beneficial to muscle tone, but the contact they provide will help you feel less isolated, and more in touch with those close to you, who share the experience. Vigorous activities such as sports, dance classes, exercise programs, or the martial arts will improve your sense of being in touch with your body.

"After I decided to start up regular aerobics classes," a man exclaimed with some surprise, "I got a sense of wholeness about my body that I never had before I learned I had been infected with AIDS!"

A physical education instructor with AIDS found that sharing his knowledge about massage and passive exercise technique had an added bonus. By providing therapy and comfort to those who were too ill to exercise on their own, he greatly increased his own feelings of self-worth. The human touch does more than soothe sore muscles, it restores a healthy sense of self as well.

Mind and Body

Over the years, each of us develops a mental image in our mind about our body. We may not be completely satisfied with that image, but we are usually more comfortable with it in the presence of someone we love who loves us in return. The reflection of our self-worth in the eyes of a loved one helps us feel physically and sexually attractive.

Feeling "infected," especially when the feeling is reinforced by actual physical problems such as hair loss, nausea, and fatigue, can certainly convince you that you are no longer physically appealing. And if you believe you are unattractive, you may anticipate rejection and avoid physical contact with your partner. Time, along with demonstrations of love, understanding, and affection by your partner and family, should help you work through feelings about your changed body image.

Sex: New Ways, Safe Ways

The problems and emotional stress of AIDS will follow you into the bedroom. Some individuals seem to handle serious financial problems and household crises with relative ease, only to find that sexual problems threaten their relationship. There are many reasons for such problems.

A few people still have the mistaken belief that HIV infection cannot be prevented. One man complained, "I'm so afraid I'll expose someone in my family. I know AIDS is not catching from casual contact, but I still sterilize everything in the bathroom every time I go in there! You can see why I would never have sex with anyone again!" Fact: HIV infection *can* be prevented. If your mate, or someone in your family believes otherwise, call your physician and counselor and arrange appointments for both of you. Sexual activity can be active and fulfilling without the exchange of body fluids that can infect.

You may feel embarrassed discussing sex or your personal sexual relationships with others, but problems with sexuality are too important to let modesty stand in the way of solutions. Keep in mind that in most cases your partner is more concerned about your well-being than his or her own. Your partner's overriding concerns probably begin with "Will the treatment work?" and "How can I show my love and support?" . . . and, only finally, "What about sex?" In reality, your partner may be afraid to appear overeager and may therefore seem to be insensitive. So it may be up to you to show whether or not you are interested in sexual activity, as well as other expressions of affection—hugging, caressing, and kissing.

Remember, it's not only the physical appearance of your body that makes you "sexy." You also have intangible qualities that your mate finds attractive. A sense of humor, intellect, a certain romantic nature, or great common sense, unique talents, and loving devotion—each of us knows what qualities in others are special or attractive to us; and it's more than anatomy. If you feel you have lost the qualities that make you attractive, counseling can help you, and your mate, restore your perspective.

For those in a relationship, infidelity, or more likely the fear of it, can present a problem. Exploring these fears with your mate is probably the best way to deal with them. If you admit that you are plagued by uncertainty and insecurity, you will probably receive the needed support and affection that will dismiss your doubts.

Some AIDS patients cite preference for a certain sexual act as the cause of sexual problems. You need to deal, not only with a realistic approach to the dangers of exposure, but with what this perceived change in your body has done to your feelings about yourself. As awkward as it may seem, you may need to find new ways to communicate sexually and verbally with your partner. An inability to express what you feel will only complicate this already difficult period.

Talk with your mate about sexual fulfillment. Experiment with ways you can still fulfill each other, without fear of exposure to infection. Approach lovemaking with the same sense of adventure that you did before you learned each other's unique desires, preferences, and "mental erogenous zones." Concentrate on the "how to," rather than the "we can't."

When You Are Down

At times, even after all your treatments and all your efforts to strengthen your body and improve your attitude, it will seem that not nearly enough is being done. Although treatment for AIDS or ARC can sometimes be very aggressive, it may be hard to see positive results. Prolonged fatigue can be debilitating. Drug treatments can extend for weeks or months, and the side effects can include nausea, hair loss, fatigue, cramps, skin discoloration, or weight loss. It is not unusual, for a short time, for treatments to cause more discomfort than the initial disease. You may find that you must contend with your emotional reactions to treatments, as well as with physical changes and side effects.

It is hard to believe that your health is improving when you feel absolutely rotten. It is hard to be hopeful when you feel even worse than you did at the time of diagnosis. The repetition of tests and treatments may seem endless. You may be convinced that there has never been a day when you didn't feel awful; there will never be one when you feel normal—if only you could remember how normal feels. Some even interpret their physical reactions to treatment as signs that the end is near. This is not at all likely to be the case, although you may have to remind yourself of this fact again and again. Feel comfortable in sharing such anxieties with your doctor and counselor.

A return to the hospital setting for new tests or additional treatment causes anxiety for some. Researchers studied a group of women undergoing radiation therapy following breast cancer surgery. They found that the women felt much better immediately after leaving the hospital than they did when follow-up treatment began. You may find it unsettling, indeed, to return again and again to the hospital or physician's office, places which may have come to represent the most frightening aspects of AIDS. Frequently it is not the treatment itself, but the symbols of change in your life that make such visits so difficult. You may not be able to change the test and treatment schedule, but there is much you can do to change your attitudes:

1. Plan special activities for the days when you feel well, ones that can be started at any time without added complications.

2. Brace yourself for the days when you feel awful by preparing your bedroom with interesting reading materials, a favorite videotape, something special to drink or eat, or anything that makes you feel pampered and comfortable.

3. Inform people that treatment may cause shifts in your mood. It's helpful to others, and easier for you, if you can let them know in a fairly matter-of-fact way that you will have up days and down days.

4. Be familiar with each side effect of treatment. The known is almost always easier to deal with than the unknown. Not only does knowledge reduce fear, but some side effects can be eliminated or at least eased through changes in treatment, in medication dosages, or in diet. There is no need to be more uncomfortable than you absolutely have to be.

The best way to obtain accurate information about your own situation is through a frank and thorough discussion with the physician or nurse administering treatment. Your doctor or treatment center should also have written materials on what to expect in the way of side effects from your treatments. Talk about your doubts and concerns when they occur. If the health professionals treating you seem unresponsive or too busy, or if your physician has been less than helpful, try one of the information resources or special support groups referred to in the previous chapter. Ask one more nurse, one more resident, one more organization for help or guidance. As one of my "expert patients" wrote, "I never stop looking for assistance whenever I need it. It's a mistake to give up when I'm ignored or treated badly by any one individual. There is always a source of information somewhere. And I'm not afraid to look for it." He is so right! There is *always* one more source for information, *and* comfort. Don't let prejudiced opinions or tactless comments dictate your approach to your personal problems.

Medical fraud and mistreatment are rare, but if you have been subjected to cruelty, or obvious malpractice, report the incident immediately in detail to the proper authorities (such as your state board of medical examiners).

Keep your mind busy. Even if you are unable to perform strenuous activity, you can still take on a challenging handicraft activity or a structured meditation technique that will leave you less time for self-pity, and help you regain your sense of purpose. Writing, composing music, painting, furniture building, sewing, and even reading aloud to others all provide opportunities for creative growth and a sense of pride. If anything needs supporting and strengthening, it is the way we feel about ourselves. Acquiring interests and developing talents can help you build that strength and self-confidence.

What Mates Can Do

Couples choosing to face AIDS together will be tested as they have never been tested before. Facing this battle together can strengthen everything that is good in a relationship. It can show how minor the problems are that were once considered so important. But AIDS can also strain to the breaking point a relationship already jeopardized by other serious problems.

Sometimes sexual expression becomes the barometer of a relationship. In a mature relationship, sex is an expression of love, affection, and respect—not the sole basis for that relationship. As one man put it, "We had a good relationship before this and there is no basis for thinking we're going to lose it all now. I don't need to use this as an excuse not to have sexual relations, and my mate doesn't need to use this as an excuse to seek a new, more exciting partner. Any real problems were there before the changes we're going through now."

If your partner has AIDS, the debilitation caused by treatments and disease can strongly affect your emotions. You expect to be able to see beyond the physical changes to the person within, to the one who more than ever needs your love, and physical reassurance of your love. Nonetheless, you might find yourself withdrawing, seemingly unable to provide that support. You might feel awkward about physical contact because you think your partner is not ready for it and you will be judged insensitive. Perhaps you are dealing with personal fears of also being exposed to disease. It helps to remember that touching, holding, hugging, and caressing are all safe ways to show that you accept what is happening and still care. Physical touch is vitally important to the person with AIDS and poses no threat to your own health. More than your words, it is your actions that tangibly show your love, that express your belief in the patient's continued desirability as a physical being.

Admittedly, it is a difficult time. Beset by reactions to treatment, anxiety, self-doubt, or a mistaken notion of what your real feelings are, your loved one may withdraw from you. It will help if you can recall ways you used to solve problems together. Your partner's insecurities have not changed the basic makeup of his personality. As you have in the past, together, you can prevent a cycle of misunderstandings from developing by openly communicating your needs and feelings. As the well partner, reach out gently and repeatedly to reassure your mate that AIDS cannot destroy your love. Keep this checklist handy when times are rough:

1. Make sure you are doing whatever you can to re-establish bonds of closeness and caring.
2. Maintain a schedule of activities that you enjoy and that give you peace of mind. Taking good care of yourself assures that you will be able to give your best to your partner.
3. If barriers grow, get professional help. A counselor can help you identify your feelings and work out your reactions

toward the patient and the disease. Ask for help before the situation gets out of hand.

4. Be honest with your partner when you feel that too much of the responsibility has been placed upon your shoulders. Ask for advice and assistance in making decisions.

5. Include in your daily routine a self-check list to make sure that you are bearing no more than your strength will allow.

6. Seek counsel and advice from friends who have already experienced what you are going through.

Most people find ways to overcome the stress that AIDS places on their relationships. They find strength in each other, and work to establish a new and comfortable routine. Sharing their feelings with each other has usually been their first step in dealing with problems. Though it may be difficult at first, communication will grow easier with time.

A trained counselor can help you understand ways in which you can begin helping each other. You should include family therapists or psychiatric social workers in your personal AIDS treatment team, and consult with them on a regular basis. You will find that support groups where couples discuss how they cope with AIDS can be helpful, especially in dealing with intimate problems. Personal barriers often fall when you know you have sympathetic and experienced confidants who can offer practical (and tested) guidance. Those who have found ways to maintain or recapture closeness and intimacy throughout the ordeal of AIDS can often help others, especially in a group setting.

Chapter 9

Opening a Window to the World

Anyone intimately affected by AIDS knows how it can change our relationships outside the family as well as those within. Friends react as they do to other difficult situations: some handle it well; others are unable to maintain any association at all. Casual acquaintances, and even strangers, can cause unintended pain by asking questions about your personal lifestyle or about obvious changes in your mental attitude or physical appearance.

Friends Who Don't Call

Lost friendships are one of the real heartbreaks people with AIDS face. Friends do not call for any number of reasons. They might not know how to respond to a change in your attitude or appearance, or to a change in their perception of you as a person. They may avoid you because they feel threatened by the possibility of your death. Or, more likely, because they have been reminded of their own mortality. Changes in friends' behavior do not necessarily mean they no longer care about you. Still, it is not very comforting to know that you have friends "out there," especially if they have so little confidence in their importance as friends that they would rather say nothing than risk saying the wrong thing.

If you believe discomfort rather than fear is keeping a particular friend from visiting, you might try a phone call to help dissolve that discomfort. Of course, you cannot overcome all the reasons why people may avoid you. Some may still believe that AIDS is contagious by casual contact; certainly, you cannot call them up and say, "Hey, get out of the Dark Ages. It's not catching!" But you can arrange for one of your more understanding friends to visit them and tactfully convey the message for you.

"I see that my friends don't know how to talk to me, and they shy away from me," wrote one person with AIDS. "Most people are very ignorant on the subject of AIDS, and they are either afraid they might find out how I got it, or, maybe worse, they'll get it too."

Knowing that others are ignorant does little to lessen the hurt and frustration of being needlessly isolated. You can only change the attitudes of others if you can talk to them. Examine carefully whether your friends are actually shunning you, or whether, perhaps, you have withdrawn from them to protect your own feelings. You can neither enlighten nor draw comfort from an empty room. If possible, the best place for you to be is out in the world with other people.

Try not to use how you feel as an excuse. You will have days when you'd just as soon "Aunt Ida" not drop in unannounced, but making your health a constant excuse to avoid social contacts may send everyone the message to stay away—particularly if "Aunt Ida" is the one who delivers the message.

Making It Easier for Others

Most people fall somewhere between staunch friends and "avoiders." Most are searching for ways to feel comfortable with your situation. They may say things that sound inane, insincere, or hurtful. You have to keep reminding yourself that they are trying their best. If you show you are willing to talk about sensitive issues, but won't dwell on ones that are too sensitive for them, they may finally relax and just be themselves.

A courageous college student, diagnosed with full-blown AIDS, explained, "No one knew I was gay. At first, before I got sick, there wasn't any pressure about it, but when I got AIDS, I knew the time was coming when I wouldn't be able to hide my being gay anymore. How could I hide my lover, who was caring for me? More important, was it worth risking a good relationship by keeping it wrapped up in white lies? So I took the chance—and I lost a few friends. But I was amazed at how many people got closer to me when they knew what I was going through; when I told them the truth. I'm not one of those who believe that there will be a time when nobody feels uneasy or thinks there's anything unusual about being gay. There will always be people who don't understand. I'm not bitter about those people. I am comfortable with myself, so I'm pretty much at ease with them, and I keep trying to make them feel at ease with me. I know some of them are afraid of me, or think that I've changed somehow, and sometimes they say some pretty stupid things. I have learned a lot about human nature by 'coming out' in a closeted world. And I'm sorry that it took AIDS to get me to this point. But I am willing, even glad, to share my feelings about being a gay male. And the number of close friends I have says to me that I made the right choice."

A man who had extensive purple discolorations on his skin, common with Kaposi's sarcoma, explained how he tried to lessen the discomfort of others without causing discomfort for himself. He focused on his "temporary" appearance, rather than on the prognosis. "Seeing the expression of shock on my friends' faces, I became determined to find some way to put them at ease. Now, if I can speak to them on the telephone before they see me for the first time, I immediately say, 'You know how you once said you'd love me even if I was polka-dotted? Well, at the moment I am!'" When asked if he felt he might be making fun of himself, he replied, "No! I find it much more frustrating to have people avoiding me or looking away from me, to try to save my feelings by pretending nothing's wrong, than just admitting that I look a lot different these days."

We can't all be that direct. He had been a straightforward man all his life. But he had let his friends know, with a sense of humor, that he still wanted to talk, despite his physical appearance.

Friends Who Want to Help

Many times friends are waiting for some clue as to what behavior is appropriate. They might not be sure you want company. They might call to "see how things are going," then add, as they hang up the phone, "Let me know if there's anything I can do to help." These friends are really asking for direction, giving you clues that they will support you if you'll only give them some guidance on how to proceed. The next time friends or relatives offer assistance, try to look at their offer in that light. If you can think of something specific they can do, one chore they can take off your hands, you have done them, and yourself, a favor.

Bob hasn't been out of the house since I got sick. I think Saturday afternoon at the flea market would do wonders for him. Would you get him out of here so I can have a little time to myself?

We'll be at the hospital most of the day tomorrow for a transfusion and tests. It would really help if you take my list and pick up a few groceries.

Ted's family is coming to visit, and we just don't have room for them all. Would you mind some company in your guest room for the weekend?

I don't feel much like talking these days, but if you'd bring your needlepoint and come sit with me, I'd sure enjoy your company.

I need some diversion. Are there any good videos out that we could watch together?

Most people are grateful if there is something concrete they can do to show their continuing friendship. If such tasks bring them into your home, it gives them a chance to see that you are alive and functioning—and not a helpless victim just wasting away. Their next visit will be easier, and soon they'll be able to drop by without a "reason."

Choosing to help friends in this way is no easy undertaking. When you feel stretched to the breaking point just keeping your own life going, it is difficult to extend your energies further to make others feel at ease. It can be a new and difficult experience for some, this reaching out, but finding that it works can be deeply fulfilling. We all feel better giving than receiving, so it might be easier if you think of your requests as giving others the chance to feel useful, rather than as simply asking for help.

You Are Not Alone

Regardless of what you do, some friends may desert you. This is a unique and frightening kind of loneliness for any human being to endure. There are no easy answers, but there is also no excuse for prolonging the time you spend alone. The mutual support of people with AIDS can provide solace and comfort. And there are still others in the community who need your support as much as you need theirs. Being housebound need not deprive you of visits from others who would feel more comfortable sharing quiet moments or deeply felt sorrow with you, knowing that you will understand. A physician, social worker, counselor, visiting nurse, or member of the clergy can help you contact other patients or shut-ins who could use company or a friendly phone call.

Don't assume that only people suffering from AIDS or other serious illnesses will spend time with you. Remember that people in perfectly good health also have problems and are sometimes lonely, too.

Preparing for Work

For many of us, work forms the cornerstone of life. It provides a measurement of self-worth, satisfaction, and a chance to interact with peers, in addition to income. Returning to work as soon as you are physically able is one way to restore stability to your life. If illness or reactions to treatment make it impossible to return to a former line of work, investigate the availability of retraining programs within your community to prepare you for other work, or watch for part-time employment opportunities that are less taxing to your limited energy.

You may find, on returning to work, that your relationships with coworkers have changed. One patient with AIDS learned that his associates had requested separate bathroom facilities for him—that old "AIDS is contagious by casual contact" myth again! Some acquaintances will make assumptions that will come as shocking surprises. A happily married heterosexual father of four, infected through a contaminated blood transfusion, returned to work and was greeted by his assistant with the news that "Even if you *are* gay, we're here to support you."

Many people face an "if we pretend no one here will ever have AIDS, it will go away" approach by coworkers, and that can be most demoralizing. You may find that if you look well, and are able to function, people tend to underestimate the seriousness of your condition. They might mumble something like, "Glad you're back; you look great," and never ask how you really feel. In turn, you might find that you resent their good health and nonchalance, and wonder what happened to the companionship you'd looked forward to in returning to work. The best you can do is assume that your coworkers, like so many others, are unsure of what to say, or are trying to protect your feelings—or their own. You may need to take the first step in opening the doors of communication.

Others returning to work may be perfectly delighted with a cavalier attitude toward their condition. "Glad you're back," may be all you want to hear before plunging into your old routine. If you are being coddled at home, returning to a situation where others do not think of you as sick might be the best therapy.

Some people believe it eases relationships with coworkers if they are quite open about their condition. One young man told the following story when he was asked why he had decided to publicly share some of his experiences in living with AIDS:

When I first was diagnosed, and after I felt well enough to go back to work, I reported to the owner of the company. (I'm in an executive sales manager position with a very large company.) Of course I had to be pretty straightforward with him and let him know that I had been diagnosed with AIDS, and that I didn't know if I could work a full day, and that if I couldn't, I needed to know where that would put me in relation to medical and health insurance, and what was going to happen in the way of my future with the company, and would my salary in fact be cut. I mean there's 50 million things that go through your mind—I don't care what level you're at. I think it's particularly difficult in an executive level when you're held under scrutiny by employees and by customers. I know it was a big concern on the owner's mind. We talked through all that and he asked, what should he do? Should he tell people and should we do this or that, and I said, "Look, if someone has enough interest to ask questions or show concern, then I think we need to be straightforward with them and tell them yes, this is what he has. I think what you, as the owner of this company, do to me, how you react to me as a person with AIDS, is going to determine how everybody else in the company and our customers handle it. If you're positive about me and you want me here as long as I can function in my job, then that's how they'll accept it." And he agreed, and it's been fine.

If AIDS treatment means leaving your old job, discrimination may be a real obstacle to finding new work. Even the person who is completely recovered from any opportunistic infections may find it difficult to obtain employment. The rationale often heard is that people who have been infected, or been diagnosed with AIDS, will take too many sick days, are poor insurance risks, or will make coworkers uncomfortable.

How do you cope? You might begin by collecting information about your legal rights and opportunities. The Rehabilitation Act of 1973, a Federal statute, includes persons who have been treated for AIDS among the handicapped, and thus you may be covered by that

Act. You may not think of yourself as handicapped, but it is indeed a handicap if misconceptions about AIDS have limited your chances of keeping your job or finding another. In substance, the Act requires firms with contracts or subcontracts to the Federal government of $50,000 or more, and with fifty or more employees, to prepare and maintain an affirmative action program for the handicapped—and that means you. (Such a program may also include rehabilitation training.) In addition, the Act makes it illegal to discriminate against a handicapped individual by any entity, regardless of size, if it receives money, in any amount, from the Department of Health and Human Services.

Today, many firms, local government offices, and educational and health institutions do business with, or receive funding from the Federal government. You might want to apply for work in such institutions first. If you applied for a job with a firm doing business with the Federal government and believe you were denied the job because of your HIV-positive status or AIDS diagnosis, you can file a complaint with the Office of Federal Contract Compliance Programs of the United States Department of Labor under section 503 of the Rehabilitation Act. If your complaint is against an agency receiving money from the Department of Health and Human Services, file your action with the DHHS Office of Civil Rights under section 504 of the Act.

You can obtain information and assistance from national and regional offices of the Rehabilitation Services Administration, the Equal Employment Opportunities Commission, the National Labor Relations Board, the American Civil Liberties Union and most labor unions. A number of states also have passed statutes prohibiting discrimination against AIDS patients and persons with HIV-positive test results. Your state department of labor or office of civil rights can advise you on the law. (The Labor Department also may be able to refer you to rehabilitation and retraining programs.)

There have been literally hundreds of "standards" written and promoted as "company policy" concerning AIDS in the workplace. The Citizens' Commission on AIDS, reflecting the World Health Organization's resolutions adopted in May of 1988, drew up the

following principles which have been endorsed by over sixty major
New York corporations.

Ten Principles for the Workplace in Response to AIDS

1. Persons with AIDS or HIV infection are entitled to the
   same rights and opportunities as people with other serious
   or life-threatening diseases.
2. Employment policies must, at a minimum, comply with
   Federal, state, and local laws and regulations.
3. Employment policies should be based on the scientific and
   epidemiological evidence that people with AIDS or HIV
   infection do not pose a risk of transmission of the virus to
   coworkers through ordinary workplace contact.
4. The highest level of management and union leadership
   should unequivocally endorse nondiscriminatory employment policies and educational programs about AIDS.
5. Employers and unions should communicate their support
   of these policies to workers in simple, clear, and unam-
   biguous terms.
6. Employers should provide employees with sensitive, accurate, and up-to-date education about risk reduction in
   their personal lives.
7. Employers have a duty to protect the confidentiality of
   employees' medical information.
8. To prevent work disruption and rejection by coworkers of
   an employee with AIDS or HIV infection, employers and
   unions should undertake education for all employees before such an incident occurs, and as needed thereafter.
9. Employers should not require HIV screening as a part of
   general pre-employment or workplace physical examinations.
10. In those special occupational settings where there may be a
    potential risk of exposure to HIV (for example, in health
    care, where workers may be exposed to blood or blood

products), employers should provide specific, ongoing education and training, as well as the necessary equipment,
to reinforce appropriate infection control procedures and
ensure that they are implemented.

Chapter 10

Choosing Life

Whatever the stage of your illness, and whether the outlook for your recovery is good or poor, the days will continue to come and go, one at a time, and patient and family must learn to live with each one. It's not easy. On learning the diagnosis, some may decide that death is inevitable, and there is nothing to do but give up and wait. Others, and they are many, somehow find the courage to live. Among them, there are some who go on to make major contributions to the world around them.

Orville Kelly, a newspaperman who suffered from an incurable form of cancer, viewed his impending death with the same loneliness, despair, and helplessness that many HIV-positive individuals today experience. He remarked that his depression continued from his first hospitalization through his first outpatient chemotherapy treatment. Yet when he at last began to talk to his wife and children about his fears and anxieties, he found he was able to turn his feelings into a newspaper article—an article that led eventually to the founding of Make Today Count, a mutual help group for people with cancer that now includes several hundred local chapters.

The heroes of the fight against AIDS number in the thousands.

Norman Redman, a British soccer referee, was suspended from refereeing because of prejudice about the potential health risk he might pose to players. Combined with the frustrations and fears facing anyone with a positive HIV status, such a blow would have defeated many in his place. Redman chose, instead, to take control of his life. He went on to file lawsuits to defend his right to work; he has since been voted Referee of the Year by the Chichester and District Sunday Football League, and been nominated for a position on the British Press Council.

Not all who are determined to wage war against AIDS will survive, but frequently those who choose to take on the obstacles as challenges leave behind rich legacies for those who follow. Patrick Haney, a man many considered a pioneer in the field of AIDS counseling, could have given up soon after his HIV-positive status was confirmed. Instead, he founded a Persons With AIDS Coalition, a now famous national AIDS support network; he cofounded IN-FORUM, one of the first AIDS information and referral agencies in Florida; and he twice testified before the AIDS Commission appointed by President Ronald Reagan, while also serving as a spokesman for the Palm Beach County Health Department in Florida.

All of us must work through our individual feelings about death, fear, and isolation in our own good time. It is hard to overcome these feelings if we have never confronted them head on, but it is a necessary, ongoing struggle. One day brings confidence and hope, and often without explanation, the next day brings despair. No one can be expected to set aside such feelings and immediately return to life as it was, nor have any of the heroes we read about done so. Yet, most people find that it helps considerably if, day by day, they strive to return to their normal lives. Each day brings pleasures and responsibilities totally outside the realities of AIDS. The days can be more valuable if you can learn to enjoy ordinary moments as well as memorable ones. This is true whether you have weeks or years left. It is true, in fact, whether you have a life-threatening disease, or not. Physical well-being is closely tied to emotional well-being. The time you take out from worrying about AIDS strengthens you for the time you must devote to it.

Places to Go and Things to Do

When you have AIDS, you need responsibilities, diversions, outings, and companionship, just as before. As long as you are able, you should go to work, take the kids to the zoo, play cards with friends, and take vacations. If you are single, and uncomfortable with the prospect of sexual relationships, keep in mind that dating need not always be a mating ritual. Persons with AIDS can and do form new relationships, just as they did before they were diagnosed with disease. If you believe that a mate or lover is not in the picture, perhaps a roommate or new confidant is. Keep the door open to new possibilities.

Try to remember that, although responsible pursuits make life meaningful, you need activities that give you pleasure as well as a sense of purpose. In fact, some people find AIDS is a call to action, to do the fun, adventurous, or out-of-the-ordinary things they've always wanted to do, but have put off as being not quite responsible. That's a great idea. It will help ward off two overreactions—giving up and trying to cram a lifetime of accomplishment into a very short time. Too often we fill up our lives with meaningful activities and neglect the frivolous outlets that keep us sane. And we tend to forget how important a sense of humor is. Being sick doesn't give us a sense of humor, but a sense of humor can certainly help get us through being sick. There is no scientific or medical proof for it, but AIDS patients who have "places to go and things to do" seem to live longer. "Life has never been fuller, and I've never felt stronger or better." A year and a half before that statement was made, this young man, who was at the time believed to be dying of *Pneumocystis* pneumonia, had been told he had only days to live.

Many have found that they cannot retire from living. They simply have too much interest in life to let go of it. "I've had to fight letting depression take over now and then," one such person declared, "but I just started this exciting new company and I want to see where this is going to go! Besides, I haven't paid all of my bills yet!"

Doing, it might be pointed out, is not the same as *over*doing. Try to recognize your limitations as well as your capabilities. Exhaustion weakens our physical and emotional defenses. Fatigue can bring on crushing despair. Many people have found that adequate rest is an excellent safeguard to fend off depression.

Pain also can make a mockery of your attempts to function normally, but much can be done to control pain without drugging the senses. Pain, especially if prolonged, should be discussed with your physician so that it can be kept to a minimum.

"Putting one's affairs in order" is a desire that strikes many who learn they have AIDS. This is not the same as giving up. In fact, everyone needs to review insurance policies, update wills, and clean out closets and drawers from time to time—and this is something constructive you can do. Family and friends should never dismiss a patient's need to discuss taking care of things "just in case." Frequently peace of mind comes from knowing that in the event of untimely death, the details have been arranged. And that is as true for those who are well as it is for those who are not.

If a discussion about taking one's own life arises, handle it with dignity and respect. Such discussions are seldom the intent to commit suicide that they appear to be. Frequently they are the product of a need to keep all options open and an appeal for support and strength.

A California man found he could not sleep because he feared he might someday suffer from AIDS. Though he had no physical symptoms of infection, he lived in daily terror that serious disability and pain might one day make his life a prolonged nightmare. When he learned of a drug available in Sweden for self-induced death, he arranged to travel there on his vacation to obtain it. When he returned home, and told his family about what he had done, they were furious with him. But two years later, his "little black pill" still rests in his jewelry box, untouched, and seldom thought about. He sleeps well, his health is good, and his only comment is "I have assurance that I can end it, if I have to, with dignity, and on my own schedule."

In most cases, having discussed issues that seem negative leaves room for positive action to follow. Organizations that have provided information and resources concerning "right to die" legislation and "no heroics" bills have helped fill a valuable need. Never underestimate the healing power of having peace of mind.

Getting Involved

It is obvious that most of these remarks have been directed toward the HIV-infected person or the patient with AIDS who is part of a family, or who has a healthy relationship from which to draw strength. Many live alone, however, and some feel they have no one to "live for." This feeling increases loneliness and can make the will to live seem a bitter irony. You may want to pull the covers up over your head and die. If you have no one else to provide encouragement, you may have to act as your own cheering squad until new friends can help you build a support system. It is hard, but not impossible. Although AIDS presents unique problems, many of the issues are like those faced by people with other life-threatening illnesses throughout history.

An amazing gentleman of 73, who had been treated on and off for eight years for Hodgkin's disease, described how he coped. "I kept on fighting. This is what you must do. Positive thinking and an active life are two things that will do a great deal to relieve the tension." In order to stay involved with life and mentally active, he enrolled in his old university and began work on his master's degree. "Some people think I'm crazy," he admits. "Maybe I am, but it's a nice crazy anyway. At least, I have achieved happiness. Can most healthy people say that?"

An elderly woman with cancer decided she wanted what time was left for her to count. She was not able to move any distance from her room, but knowing the feeling of intense cold that often bothered her, she decided to make lap robes for nursing homes. She said, "I know what it is to shake with cold and so I started knitting. Those old folks were so excited to get a new blanket that I just kept going.

Now I'm making doll clothes for their grandchildren, fixing toys, and just don't seem to have enough time to do all the things I love to do. I never waste time worrying about tomorrow."

Not everyone can go beyond himself and give to others to this extent. You may not have the physical or emotional strength. It may not feel natural to your personality, and you are still the same person you were. But many find AIDS is easier to live with if they choose constructive ways to fill their time—to make at least part of each day count for what they can put into it.

Support Means Respect

The desire to "do something, anything," is common to nearly everyone with a family member or close friend who has AIDS. There is probably very little you can do to change the course of AIDS, so you do everything you can for the person. Sometimes, doing everything is the worst course to follow.

People with AIDS still have the same needs, and often the same capabilities, as they did before. If they are physically able, they need to participate in their normal range of activities and responsibilities—from buying a new house, right down to taking out the garbage. Helplessness, or worse, an unnecessary feeling of helplessness, is one of the greatest trials for the person with AIDS. In the words of one:

> I am angry about the way people with AIDS are automatically treated as if we were mentally incompetent. Our relatives have rights: we have none. This is by a sort of mutual consent, an unconscious conspiracy which seems to be part of our culture. Let an individual become a patient and he is judged, without any 'competency hearing,' as if he had been found to be incompetent in a court of law. Only the relatives are consulted or empowered to make decisions.

This man's words stand as a lesson to us all. Although bedridden, a patient is more often than not still able to discuss treatment options, financial arrangements, the children's school problems, and what color to paint the bedroom. The rest of the family must make every effort to preserve, as much as possible, the patient's dignity and customary role within the family. The least you can do is keep the patient informed of necessary decisions. You can help the seriously ill patient ward off feelings of helplessness or abandonment if you continue to share your activities, goals, and dreams, as before.

A patient with severe fatigue commented, "I get frustrated because I've always been so independent. That changes. You have to let people start doing things for you. And, well, I'm just starting to ask—it's been over a year and I'm just starting to ask, like calling people and saying I need a baby-sitter so that Dan can go and do something for so many hours. If you keep some humor to it, it really helps."

Few who are well know what it is like to be placed in a position of dependency. AIDS not only threatens your life, but attacks your sense of self, as a whole person, as well. Feelings of helplessness are real enough when you are flat on your back. Family and friends must make every effort not to compound the stress, by ignoring the wishes of the patient, or worse, by trying to make an invalid of a person who is able to function on his own.

Staying on Track

The needs of the family are important. The family should maintain normal living patterns, as much as possible. This is important for long-range as well as day-to-day coping. Sometimes, when the patient is in active treatment, family life becomes totally disrupted by the uncertainty of whether good or bad times are ahead. When that happens, it can be harder to resume functioning as a unit during periods of extended remission and a return to good health.

"My most surprising emotional problem," a patient reported, "was finding that my improved health and ability to get up and do things spoiled the plans that everyone had made for themselves. Things they thought they couldn't do while I was so sick were scheduled for days when I would be more stable, but now that I have a surprisingly good day, one that nobody expected, it's too late to be included. I don't want them to stay home on my account, but I know they will anyway."

Understanding the possibility of such a situation might help prevent it. There are many ways we cope with fear, anxiety and the threat of loss or death. One unfortunate, but common, way is to begin preparing for an event by thinking about it, without being aware that we are doing so, as if it had already happened. Thus, we "rehearse" life as it will be, so that we can assume our new roles more easily when the time comes. Sadly, when a family member has AIDS, we may begin "rehearsing" the future in our minds. We may begin to "practice" how the family will function if that loved one dies. Watch for signs that you are excluding the patient, and turn your routine back to normal if you are. Knowing that these things can happen, however, try not to feel guilty if you find yourself emotionally out of step with remission or recovery.

From Now On

Abraham Lincoln once commented, "It has been my observation that people are just about as happy as they make up their minds to be." Happiness and peace of mind are certainly devastated by the news of AIDS, and AIDS is not something anyone forgets. Anxious moments return as active treatment and the waiting begin. A cold, a cramp, or an unexplained bruise may be cause for panic. As regular checkups approach, or reports on immune response are received, you swing between hope and despair. You watch for news of the elusive breakthrough or cure and you may find you feel more anxious than hopeful.

No one expects you to forget, or remove from your mind, that you have been infected with HIV, that you may develop AIDS, or that your health may change, often in subtle ways. You, like your family and loved ones, must cope with the insecurity of not knowing the true state of your health. But, the best prescription for happiness and a sense of purpose seems to be a combination of three things: challenging responsibilities that make use of a full range of skills, activities that seek to fill the needs of others, and a generous dose of frivolity and laughter. Finding the mental discipline to "decide to fight," to stay interested and interesting, and to seek personal fulfillment in the face of adversity, all of these have made up the "pioneer spirit" of peoples throughout recorded history. Those who personally fight the battles of AIDS are most certainly such pioneers, living the unknown with incredible resolve and inner fortitude.

You will have moments when you feel you are living in the path of a tornado. Such feelings will sneak up without warning. But they will appear less often if you fill your mind with thoughts of other things than AIDS.

You may feel that your visions of the future are lost forever, and it is true that AIDS has robbed you of that blissful ignorance that once led you to believe you would live forever. But in exchange, you are granted the vision to see each day as a precious gift to use wisely and with purpose. Nothing can take that away.

Glossary

Listed below are the scientific and technical terms you will most likely encounter in learning about HIV infection, AIDS, and ARC.

ABSOLUTE HELPER T-CELL COUNT. The actual number of Helper T-cells in the blood, which is significantly lower in people whose immune systems have been affected by HIV. *See* HELPER T-CELL; HIV; CD.

ACQUIRED. Not inherited.

AIDS: Acquired Immune Deficiency Syndrome. A syndrome characterized by opportunistic infections and malignancies that arise from the severe breakdown of the body's immune system caused by HIV infection. *See* OPPORTUNISTIC INFECTION; KAPOSI'S SARCOMA (KS); HIV.

AIDS-RELATED COMPLEX. *See* ARC.

ANTIBIOTIC. A soluble substance, sometimes derived from a mold, that inhibits the growth of other organisms and is used to combat disease due to infection.

ANTIBODY. A protein made by the body during the humoral immune (B-cell) response to an infection. Antibodies "coat" foreign microbes for engulfment by white blood cells and otherwise help to destroy or to neutralize these microbes.

ANTIGEN. Any substance that provokes an immune response when introduced into the body.

ARC. AIDS-Related Complex. A complex of conditions, signs, or symptoms caused by HIV infection, including fever, unusual weight loss, prolonged fatigue, enlarged lymph nodes, and diarrhea; but *excluding* opportunistic infections and malignancies diagnostic of full-blown AIDS. *See* AIDS.

ASYMPTOMATIC INFECTION. An infection, or phase of an infection, that is without symptoms.

BACTERIUM. A microscopic single-celled plant lacking chlorophyll. Many bacteria can cause disease in man.

B-CELLS. A lymphocyte that participates in the humoral immune response of specialized immunity. B-cells destroy or neutralize foreign microbes through the production of antibodies. *See* SPECIALIZED IMMUNITY; ANTIBODY; LYMPHOCYTE.

BONE MARROW. Soft tissue located in the center of the bones and responsible for producing all blood cells after birth.

CANDIDA. A yeast that normally lives in the intestines, but that can flourish in other parts of the body when the immune system is suppressed.

CELLULAR IMMUNITY. *See* SPECIALIZED IMMUNITY.

CD. Cluster (or Common) Designation. A system of nomenclature, first devised in 1984, that labels identifying surface structures on the various types of white blood cells. CD4 is the name given to the identifying surface structure present on the Helper T-cell, and CD8, is the name given to the identifying surface structure on the killer (cytotoxic) T-cell and the suppressor T-cell.

CD4. Also called T4. *See* HELPER T-CELL; CD.

CD8. Also called T8. *See* KILLER T-CELL; SUPPRESSOR T-CELL; CD.

CLINICAL DIAGNOSIS. A diagnosis determined by signs and symptoms alone; based on subjective information (e.g., pain) and objective information (e.g., fever).

CMV. *See* CYTOMEGALOVIRUS.

CRYPTOCOCCOSIS. An infectious, airborne disease, sometimes seen in AIDS patients, caused by the fungus *Cryptococcus neoformans*. Cryptococcosis focuses primarily in the lungs, characteristically spreads to the meninges (the lining of the brain and spinal cord), and may also spread to the kidneys and skin.

CRYPTOSPORIDIOSIS. An infection, often seen in AIDS patients, caused by a protozoan parasite found in the intestines of animals. Once transmitted to man (by direct contact with the infected animal), it lodges in the intestines and causes severe diarrhea. It can be spread from person to person.

CYTOMEGALOVIRUS (CMV). A Herpes-like virus that normally infects more than half the population without any symptoms. CMV infection, often seen in AIDS patients, may result in mild flu-like symptoms of aching, fever, sore throat, weakness, and enlarged lymph nodes; or in severe cases, may cause hepatitis, mononucleosis, retinitis, and pneumonia, especially in immune-suppressed people. CMV is "shed" in body fluids, such as urine, semen, saliva, feces, and sweat.

CYTOTOXIC T-CELL. See KILLER T-CELL.

DEFINITIVE DIAGNOSIS. A diagnosis that confirms or verifies the nature or origin of an illness. Often a specific and sensitive laboratory test is necessary to establish a definitive diagnosis.

DIAGNOSIS. See CLINICAL DIAGNOSIS; DEFINITIVE DIAGNOSIS; DIFFERENTIAL DIAGNOSIS; LABORATORY DIAGNOSIS; PRESUMPTIVE DIAGNOSIS.

DIFFERENTIAL DIAGNOSIS. Comparison of symptoms and signs of similar diseases to determine which disease is most likely causing the health problem. Usually, a specific laboratory test is required to rule out one disease or the other.

DISEASE. Any abnormal condition or structure of the body resulting in a characteristic set of symptoms and signs.

DNA. Deoxyribonucleic Acid. A complex protein that is the chemical basis for heredity and the warehouse for genetic information.

EIA. See ELISA (EIA).

ELISA (EIA). Enzyme Linked Immunosorbent Assay. An established laboratory technique for the detection of antibodies to viruses in blood or serum. In HIV testing, the test does not diagnose AIDS, or detect HIV in the blood, but does indicate that infection with HIV may have occurred.

EPIDEMIOLOGY. The systematic study of the frequency and distribution of diseases within a population to determine how diseases are caused and how they are transmitted.

EPSTEIN-BARR VIRUS (EBV). A Herpes-like virus that causes one of two kinds of mononucleosis. (The other is caused by CMV.) EBV lodges in the nose and throat and is transmitted by intimate contact, for example, by kissing. It lies dormant in the lymph nodes and has been associated with Burkitt's lymphoma, a cancer of the lymph nodes. EBV is the clearest link to date between viruses and cancer.

FALSE NEGATIVE TEST RESULT. A negative test result that *falsely* indicates the absence of a certain disease in an individual who *has* that disease. In HIV testing, this usually occurs when an individual is tested *before* sufficient time has passed for HIV antibodies (which testing can detect) to be produced. False negative test results occur with both the ELISA and the Western blot.

FALSE POSITIVE TEST RESULT. A positive test result that *falsely* indicates the presence of a disease in an individual who does *not* have that disease. For example, an individual may have a positive ELISA test result for HIV and still not be infected. The ELISA is more likely to give a false positive test result for HIV than the Western blot, which does so only rarely.

FUNGUS. Member of a class of relatively primitive plants lacking chlorophyll that includes mushrooms, yeasts, rusts, molds, and smuts.

HELPER T-CELL. A lymphocyte and the single most important cell in the specialized immune response. Helper T-cells induce, help, and coordinate, the specialized immune response, which cannot function without them. The helper T-cell has an identifying surface structure called CD4 or T4. *See* CD.

HELPER-TO-SUPPRESSOR RATIO. The ratio of helper T-cells to suppressor-killer T-cells.

HIV. Human Immunodeficiency Virus. The retrovirus identified as the cause of AIDS and ARC; any of the many strains of this highly mutable virus.

HUMORAL IMMUNITY. A response of specialized immunity that produces specific antibodies against foreign organisms or substances. Humoral immune defense cells (B-cells) are lymphocytes found in the lymph and throughout the body fluids. *See* SPECIALIZED IMMUNITY.

HTLV. Human T-cell Lymphotropic Virus, or Human T-cell Leukemia-Lymphoma Virus. Any of a group of retroviruses associated with leukemias or lymphomas (HTLV-I and HTLV-II) and with Acquired Immune Deficiency Syndrome (HTLV-III and HTLV-IV).

HTLV-III. Human T-cell Lymphotropic Virus, III. A former name for HIV. *See* HTLV; HIV.

IMMUNE DEFICIENCY. A defect in immunity which may be inherited or acquired later in life. *See* NATURAL IMMUNITY; SPECIALIZED IMMUNITY.

IMMUNE SYSTEM; IMMUNITY. *See* NATURAL IMMUNITY; SPECIALIZED IMMUNITY.

IMMUNOSUPPRESSION. A process that blocks or impairs the immune system's defenses. Immunosuppression may be caused by a drug, poor nutrition, an organism, or factors yet unknown.

INCUBATION PERIOD. The interval between initial exposure to a virus or other pathogen and the appearance of the first symptom or sign of infection, during which antibodies are usually produced.

INFECTION. Invasion and reproduction of microbes in body tissues or cells, which may be symptomatic (cause disease) or asymptomatic.

KAPOSI'S SARCOMA (KS): A tumor of the walls of blood vessels, usually appearing as pink to purple, painless spots on the skin but may also occur internally with or without skin lesions. KS may be fatal if it spreads to major organs. Originally seen as a slow-growing, benign lesion in elderly men or in inhabitants of equatorial Africa.

KILLER T-CELL: A type of T-cell, also called cytotoxic T-cell, that destroys infected host cells as a function of the cellular immune response. The killer T-cell has an identifying surface structure called CD8 or T8. *See* CD.

KS. *See* KAPOSI'S SARCOMA.

LABORATORY DIAGNOSIS. Use of one or more laboratory tests to help establish or confirm a clinical diagnosis. *See* CLINICAL DIAGNOSIS.

LAS. *See* LAV.

LAV. Lymphadenopathy Associated Virus. A former name for HIV. So called because of its association with Lymphadenopathy Syndrome (LAS): A chronic enlargement of the lymph nodes resulting from HIV infection and included under the term ARC.

LESION. A general term to describe an area of altered tissue, such as an infected patch or sore in a skin disease.

LEUKOCYTE. Any white blood cell.

LYMPH NODE. Small bean-sized organ of the immune system, widely distributed throughout the body and containing lymphocytes (B-cells and T-cells).

LYMPHOCYTE. A small white blood cell, normally present in blood, lymph, and lymphatic tissue, that bears the major responsibility for carrying out the functions of the specialized immune response.

LYMPHOMA. A cancer of the lymphocytes, affecting the lymph nodes or the spleen.

LYMPHOTROPIC. Having a special affinity for lymphocytes, such as HIV has for helper T-cells.

MACROPHAGE. *See* MONOCYTE.

MICROBE. A tiny form of life, such as a protozoan, bacterium, or virus, often capable of causing disease.

MONOCYTE. A white blood cell that participates in the natural immune response and is characterized by a round nucleus without lobes. When transported to the tissues by the blood, it becomes a macrophage, which means "big eater."

NATURAL IMMUNITY. Also called Natural Immune Response. The immune system's first line of defense against foreign microbes, in which certain white blood cells destroy these microbes before they can invade or infect the body. Cells participating in this immune response are the polymorphonuclear leucocytes (polys) and the monocytes or macrophages.

OPPORTUNISTIC INFECTION. An infection that ordinarily does not cause disease in healthy persons but only in persons whose immune systems are suppressed or impaired. *Pneumocystis carinii* pneumonia is a common opportunistic infection in persons with AIDS.

PCP. *See* PNEUMOCYSTIS CARINII PNEUMONIA

PNEUMOCYSTIS CARINII PNEUMONIA (PCP): An opportunistic lung infection in people with impaired immune systems. PCP is caused by a primitive, single-celled organism, possibly a protozoan, that is normally destroyed by healthy immune systems. *See* OPPORTUNISTIC INFECTION.

POLY. *See* POLYMORPHONUCLEAR LEUCOCYTE.

POLYMORPHONUCLEAR LEUCOCYTE. A white blood cell, also called a "poly," that participates in the natural immune response and is characterized by a polylobated (many lobed) nucleus.

PRESUMPTIVE DIAGNOSIS. A preliminary diagnosis based on clinical signs and symptoms that are strongly suggestive—but not conclusive—evidence of a disease.

PROPHYLAXIS. Any substance or steps taken to preserve health or to prevent disease (e.g., Vitamin C, vaccines).

PROTOZOAN. A primitive, single-celled, free-living microbe. There are a number of protozoa that can cause disease in man, including an amoeba that causes dysentery. *Pneumocystis carinii* may also be a protozoan, although this is not certain. *See* PNEUMOCYSTIS CARINII PNEUMONIA (PCP).

REMISSION. A lessening of the severity or duration of symptoms, or their abatement altogether over a period of time.

RETROVIRUS. An RNA-virus containing the enzyme reverse transcriptase, which allows it to reverse the normal genetic sequence—to go backwards (retro = backwards)—from RNA to DNA, instead of from DNA to RNA. HIV is a retrovirus.

REVERSE TRANSCRIPTASE. An enzyme found in retrovirus (retro = backwards) that allows the normal genetic sequence to go in reverse (backwards) from RNA to DNA, instead of from DNA to RNA.

RNA. Ribonucleic acid. In normal, metabolically complete cells DNA is used to form RNA, and RNA to form the proteins needed to maintain life. *See* DNA.

SENSITIVITY. In testing, the degree to which a test can *detect* the presence of a particular disease or infection in those being tested. For example, if a test is 100% sensitive for detecting a certain disease, *all* persons with the disease will give a positive test result. High sensitivity in testing is especially important when the consequences of *failing* to detect a disease would be serious.

SEROPOSITIVE. A test result indicating that infection with a disease has occurred and that antibodies to the disease are present in the blood.

SERONEGATIVE. A test result indicating that antibodies to a disease are currently not in sufficient TITER to be detected, or that infection with the disease has not occurred.

SPECIALIZED IMMUNITY. Also called Specialized Immune Response. Immunity or resistance to a disease as a result of having protective antibodies or killer T-cells against microbes causing that disease. The immune system's second line of defense against foreign microbes, in which certain white blood cells destroy these microbes after they have invaded or infected the body. The cells that participate in this immune response are the lymphocytes: T-cells (cellular immune response) and B-cells (humoral immune response).

SPECIFICITY. In testing, the degree to which a test can *confirm* the presence of infection in an individual with a positive test result. For example, if a test is 100% specific for a certain disease, *all* persons testing positive will *actually* have that disease.

STD. Sexually Transmitted Disease. Sometimes referred to as Sexually Transmissible Disease.

SUPPRESSOR T-CELL. A lymphocyte that down-regulates or suppresses the specialized immune response (both humoral and cellular). The suppressor T-cell has the same identifying surface structure, called CD8 or T8 as the killer T-cell. Standard lymphocyte typing does not therefore distinguish between suppressor T-cells and killer T-cells. *See* CD.

SYMPTOMATIC. A state of infection associated with manifestations that are either subjective (pain), or objective (fever, weight loss).

SYNDROME. A group of symptoms or signs that together characterize a specific condition.

T-CELL. A lymphocyte, programmed by the thymus, that participates in the cellular immune response and in the overall regulation of specialized immunity. There are three types of T-cells: killer T-cells, suppressor T-cells, and helper T-cells. *See* LYMPHOCYTE; SPECIALIZED IMMUNITY; KILLER T-CELL; SUPPRESSOR T-CELL; HELPER T-CELL; LYMPHOCYTE.

THRUSH. A fungal infection of the mouth caused by Candida (a yeast); common in people with AIDS or ARC.

TITER. A laboratory measurement of the amount of something in solution; for example, of antibodies in blood.

TOXOPLASMOSIS. A disease, seen frequently in people with AIDS, caused by infection with the protozoan *Toxoplasma gondii*, often resulting in focal encephalitis (inflammation of the brain).

VIRUS. An incomplete, submicroscopic organism that cannot survive or reproduce itself outside a living cell. Viruses are composed of genetic material (DNA *or* RNA) and other proteins, surrounded by an outer covering. Many can cause disease in man. *See* HIV; RETROVIRUS.

WESTERN BLOT. A confirmatory test for antibodies to HIV; more specific and accurate than the ELISA test.

WHITE BLOOD CELL. *See* LYMPHOCYTE; POLYMORPHONUCLEAR LEUCO-CYTE; MONOCYTE.

Information and
Advocacy Resources

Across the country, AIDS advocacy groups are growing both in number and diversity. Organizations providing AIDS information can furnish you with names, addresses, and phone numbers of groups in your area.

Advocacy organizations form alliances at all levels with powerful lobbying and special interest groups to influence legislation affecting the many issues of AIDS, including housing, long-term care, medical financing and reimbursement, and community-based health care delivery.

To be effective, however, advocacy, education, and "political risk reduction" initiatives must be ongoing and sustained. They require the time, effort and financial support of all who can assist in any way.

Those who have only limited resources, or who are physically unable to put in long hours of volunteer work, can still make a major contribution by writing letters, making telephone calls, and processing newsletters. Sustained advocacy requires that educational materials be made available to all segments of the community as frequently as possible.

The following lists of organizations were compiled over a period of more than three years, and were made possible through the invaluable assistance of the Centers for Disease Control, the American Foundation for AIDS Research (AmFAR), the Public Health Service, the National Health Institute, the National AIDS Information Clearing House, and the American Medical Association, as well as of private individuals, persons with AIDS, physicians, and public health officials. The lists are by no means exhaustive, but should serve as good starting points in your search for information and referral. The organizations listed will be happy to suggest additional ways in which you can contribute to these vital programs.

AIDS Action Council
729 Eighth Street S.E., Suite 200
Washington, D.C. 20003
202-547-3101

AIDS Education Bureau
9504 Wallingford Drive
Burke, VA 22015
703-323-5777

American Civil Liberties Union Foundation
132 West 43rd Street
New York, NY 10036
212-944-9800

American Foundation for AIDS Research (AmFAR)
40 West 57th Street
New York, NY 10019
212-333-3118

American Red Cross
National Headquarters
AIDS Education Office
1730 D Street, NW
Washington, D.C. 20006
202-737-8300

Arizona Diversified Counseling Services
P.O. Box 35145
Tucson, AZ 85740

Centers for Disease Control
AIDS Information Office
Atlanta, GA 30333
404-329-2891

Citizens Commission on AIDS
for New York City and Northern New Jersey
51 Madison Avenue: Room 3008
New York, NY 10010

Coalition of Hispanic Health and Human Services Organizations
(COSSMHO)
1030 15th Street NW
Washington, D.C. 20005
202-371-2100

Gay Men's Health Crisis
Box 274
132 West 24th Street
New York, NY 10011
212-807-7517

George Washington University
Intergovernmental Health Policy Project
2011 I Street, NW: Suite 200
Washington, D.C. 20006

Hemlock Society
P.O. Box 66218
Los Angeles, CA 90066-0218
213-391-1871

Lambda Legal Defense and Education Fund
666 Broadway
New York, NY 10012
212-995-8585

National AIDS Hotline
800-342-AIDS

National AIDS Information Clearing House
P.O. Box 6003
Rockville, MD 20850
800-458-5231

National AIDS Network (NAN)
1012 14th Street, NW: Suite 601
Washington, D.C. 20005
202-347-0390

National Association of People with AIDS (NAPWA)
2025 I Street, NW: Suite 415
Washington, D.C. 20006
202-347-1317

National Gay and Lesbian Task Force
1517 U Street, NW
Washington, D.C. 20009
202-332-6483

National Gay Rights Advocates
540 Castro Street
San Francisco, CA 94114
415-863-9156

National Hemophilia Foundation
SoHo Building
110 Greene Street: Room 406
New York, NY 10012
212-219-8180

National Leadership Coalition on AIDS
1150 17th Street: Suite 202
Washington, D.C. 20036
202-429-0930

National Minority AIDS Council
P.O. Box 28574
Washington, D.C. 20038
202-544-1076

New York City Parents and Friends
of Lesbian and Gay Men, Inc.
P.O. Box 553, Lenox Hill Station
New York, NY 10021
212-463-0629

Universal Fellowship of Metropolitan Community Churches
5300 Santa Monica Boulevard: Suite 304
Los Angeles, CA 90029
213-464-5100

U.S. Council of Mayors
AIDS Program
Fourth Floor
1620 Eye Street, NW
Washington, D.C. 20006
202-293-7330

State Agencies and Hotline Services

Alabama Department of Health
AIDS Program
State Office Building, Room 662
434 Monroe Street
Montgomery, AL 36130
205-261-5017
800-228-0469

Alaska Department of Health
AIDS Health Program
3601 C Street
Anchorage, AK 99524
907-561-4406

Arizona Department of Health
Office of Health Education
431 North 24th Street
Phoenix, AZ 85008
602-230-5836
800-334-1540

Arkansas Department of Health
AIDS Activities
4815 West Markham
Little Rock, AR 72205
501-661-2135
800-445-7720

California Department of Health
Office of AIDS
P.O. Box 160146
Sacramento, CA 95816
916-445-0553
800-367-2437

Colorado Department of Health
AIDS Education Risk Reduction
Program
4210 East 11th Street
Denver, CO 80220
303-331-8320

Connecticut Department of Health
AIDS Program
150 Washington Street
Hartford, CT 06112
203-566-5058
203-566-1157

Delaware Department of Health
and Social Services
AIDS Program Office
3000 Newport Gap Pike
Building G
Wilmington, DE 19808
302-995-8422

D.C. Commission of Public Health
Division of AIDS Education
1875 Connecticut Avenue, NW
Room 838-C
Washington, DC 20009
202-673-3425
202-332-AIDS

Florida Department of Health-
Rehabilitation
Health Education and Risk
Reduction
1317 Winewood Boulevard
Building 6, Room 453
Tallahassee, FL 32399
904-487-2478
800-FLA-AIDS

Georgia Department of Human
Resources
STD Control Program
878 Peachtree Street NE
Atlanta, GA 30309
404-894-5147
800-551-2728

Hawaii Department of Health
Public Health Education
3627 Kilauea Avenue
Honolulu, HI 96816
808-735-5303
808-922-1313

Idaho Department of Health
and Welfare
AIDS Program
450 West State Street
Boise, ID 83720
208-334-5930

Illinois Department of Health
Health Education
525 West Jefferson
Springfield, IL 62761
217-782-2016
800-243-2438

Indiana Department of Health
Office of AIDS Activity
1330 West Michigan
Indianapolis, IN 46206
317-633-8406

Iowa Department of Public Health
AIDS Education
Lucas Building; Third Floor
Des Moines, IA 50319
515-281-4938
800-532-3301

Kansas Department of Health and
Environment
Office of Health Education
Forbes Field Bldg. 321; Room 13
Topeka, KS 66620
913-296-5587
800-232-0040

Kentucky Department for
Health Services
AIDS Health Education
275 East Main Street
Frankfort, KY 40621
502-564-4804
800-654-AIDS

Louisiana Office of Prevention
Medicine and Public Health
Services
325 Loyola Avenue; Room 615
New Orleans, LA 70012
504-568-5005
800-999-4379

Maine Bureau of Health
Office on AIDS
Station House, Station 11
Augusta, ME 04333
207-289-3591
800-851-AIDS

Maryland Department of Health
and Mental Hygiene Epidemiology
201 West Preston Street
Baltimore, MD 21201
301-225-6707
800-638-6252

Massachusetts Department of
Public Health
AIDS Health Education
150 Tremont Street
Boston, MA 02111
617-727-0368
800-235-2331

Michigan Department of Health
Special Office of AIDS Prevention
3423 North Logan
Lansing, MI 48909
517-335-8371
800-872-AIDS

Minnesota Department of Health
AIDS Program
717 SE Delaware Street
Minneapolis, MN 55440
612-623-5414
800-248-AIDS

Mississippi Department of Health
AIDS Education Program
P.O. Box 1700
Jackson, MS 39215
601-960-7725
800-826-2961

Missouri Department of Health
AIDS Program
P.O. Box 570
Jefferson City, MO 65102
314-751-6438

Montana Department of Health
and Environmental Services
AIDS Program
Cogswell Building
Helena, MT 59260
406-444-2457

Nebraska Department of Health
AIDS Prevention Program
P.O. Box 95007
Lincoln, NE 68509
402-471-2937
800-782-2437

Nevada State Health Division
Department of Human Resources
505 East King Street, Room 200
Carson City, NV 89710
702-885-4800

New Hampshire Department of
Health and Welfare
6 Hazen Drive
Concord, NH 03301
603-271-4490

New Jersey Department of Health
AIDS Division
363 West State Street
Trenton, NJ 08625
609-984-6000
800-624-2377

New Mexico Department of Health
and Environment Epidemiology
P.O. Box 968
Santa Fe, NM 87504
505-827-0086

New York State Department
of Health
AIDS Institute
1315 Empire State Plaza
25th Floor, Room 2580
Albany, NY 12237
518-474-8160
800-462-1884

North Carolina Health Department
AIDS Control Program
P.O. Box 2091
Raleigh, NC 27602
919-733-3419

North Dakota Department
of Health
AIDS Project
State Capitol Building
Bismark, ND 58505
701-224-8378
800-592-1861

Ohio Department of Health
AIDS Activity Unit
246 North High Street
Columbus, OH 43266
614-466-5480
800-332-AIDS

Oklahoma Department of Health
STD Division
P.O. Box 53551
Oklahoma City, OK 73152
405-271-5601

Oregon Department of Health
AIDS Program
1400 Southwest 5th Street
Room 710
Portland, OR 97201
503-229-5792

Pennsylvania Department of Health
Disease Control
P.O. Box 90
Harrisburg, PA 17108
717-787-3350
800-692-7254

Puerto Rico Department of Health
Call Box STD
Caparra Heights Station
San Juan, PR 00922
809-754-8118

Rhode Island Department of
Health
AIDS Control Program
75 Davis; Room 105
Providence, RI 02908
401-277-2362
401-277-6502

South Carolina Department
of Health
AIDS Project
2600 Bull Street
Columbia, SC 29201
803-734-5482
800-322-AIDS

South Dakota Department
of Health
AIDS Program
523 East Capital
Pierre, SD 57501
605-773-3357
800-472-2180

Tennessee Department of Health
and Environment-Disease Control
100 9th Avenue, North
Nashville, TN 37219
615-741-7387
800-342-AIDS

Texas Department of Health
Epidemiology-Health Promotion
100 West 49th Street
Austin, TX 78756
512-458-7405

Utah Department of Health
Epidemiology
288 North, 1460 West
P.O. Box 16660
Salt Lake City, UT 84116
801-538-6191
801-466-9976
800-843-9388

Vermont Department of Health
AIDS Education
60 Main Street
P.O. Box 70
Burlington, VT 05402
802-863-7245
800-882-AIDS

Virgin Islands Department
of Health
AIDS Committee
P.O. Box 7309
St. Thomas, VI 00801
809-776-8311

Virginia Department of Health
AIDS Activity Program
109 Governor Street
Room 722
Richmond, VA 23219
804-786-6267
800-533-4148

Washington Department of Health
Epidemiology-AIDS Program
1610 Northeast 150th Street
Seattle, WA 98155
206-361-2888

West Virginia Department
of Health
151 11th Avenue
South Charleston, WV 25303
304-348-5358
800-624-8244

Wisconsin Department of Health
and Social Services
AIDS Program
1 West Wilson Street
P.O. Box 309
Madison, WI 53701
608-267-5287
800-334-AIDS

Wyoming Division of Health and
Medical Services
AIDS Program
Hathaway Building
4th Floor
Cheyenne, WY 82002
307-777-7953

Suggested Reading

Badgley, Laurence, M.D. *Healing AIDS Naturally.* San Bruno, CA: Human Energy Press, 1986.

Black, Claudia. *It'll Never Happen to Me.* New York: MacMillan, 1982.

Branden, Nathaniel. *The Psychology of Self-Esteem.* New York: Bantam Books, 1969.

Carnes, Patrick. *Out of the Shadows—Understanding Sexual Addiction.* Minneapolis: CompCare Publications, 1983.

Carnes, Patrick. *Contrary to Love, Understanding Sexual Addiction. Part 2; Helping the Sexual Addict.* Minneapolis: CompCare Publications, 1985.

Colgrove, Melba, Harold H. Bloomfield and Peter McWilliams. *How to Survive the Loss of a Love.* New York: Bantam Books, 1981.

Clarkhuff, Robert R. *The Act of Helping.* Amherst, MA: Human Resource Development Press, 1983.

Hay, Louise. *You Can Heal Your Life.* Santa Monica, CA: Hay House, 1984.

Hay, Louise. *Love Your Body.* Santa Monica, CA: Hay House, 1972.

Hay, Louise. *Heal Your Body.* Santa Monica, CA: Hay House, 1984.

Johnson, Bern E. *I'll Quit Tomorrow.* San Francisco: Harper & Row, 1980.

Kirschmann, John D. and Lavon J. Dunne. *Nutrition Almanac: Second Edition.* New York: McGraw-Hill Book Company, 1984.

Kreis, Bernadine and Alice Pattie. *Up From Grief: Patterns of Recovery.* San Francisco: Harper & Row, 1969.

Kubler-Ross, Elisabeth. *Living With Death and Dying.* New York: Collier Books, 1970.

Kubler-Ross, Elisabeth. *On Death and Dying.* New York: Collier Books, 1969.

Lasch, Christopher. *The Culture of Narcissism.* New York: Warner Books, 1979.

Peck, Scott, M.D. *The Road Less Traveled.* New York: Simon & Schuster (A Touchstone Book), 1980.

Peele, Stanton, and Archie Brodsky. *Love and Addiction.* New York: New American Library, 1975.

Serinus, Jason. *Psychoimmunity & the Healing Process.* Berkeley, CA: Celestial Arts, 1986.

Shilts, Randy. *And the Band Played On.* New York: St. Martin's Press, 1987.

Tatelbaum, Judy. *The Courage to Grieve.* New York: Harper & Row, 1980.

Tavris, Carol. *ANGER: The Misunderstood Emotion.* New York: Simon & Schuster (A Touchstone Book), 1982.

U.S. Department of Health and Human Services. *Coping With AIDS.* Rockville, MD: National Institutes of Mental Health, 1986.

Medical References

Adler, M. W. "Care for patients with HIV infection and AIDS." *British Medical Journal* 295:27–30(1987).

American Medical Association. AIDS Board of Trustees. "Prevention and control of acquired immunodeficiency syndrome. An interim report." *Journal of the American Medical Association* 258:2097–2103(1987).

American Medical Association. Council on Scientific Affairs and AIDS Panel. *AIDS: Information on AIDS for the Practicing Physician.* Chicago: American Medical Association, 1987.

Barnes, D. M. "New questions about AIDS test accuracy." *Science* 238: 884–885(1988).

Broder, S. "Pathogenic human retroviruses." *New England Journal of Medicine* 318:243–245(1988).

Centers for Disease Control. *Fact about AIDS.* Washington, D.C.: U.S. Government Printing Office, 1988. (G.P.O. 532–013–1988).

Centers for Disease Control. *Human Immunodeficiency Virus (HIV) Infection Codes: Official Authorized Addendum ICD–9–CM* (Effective January 1, 1988). *Morbidity and Mortality Weekly Report* 36(S–7):1–24(1987).

Centers for Disease Control. "Human immunodeficiency virus infection in the United States." *Morbidity and Mortality Weekly Report* 36(49):1–30(1987).

Friedland, G. H., and R. S. Klein. "Transmission of the human immunodeficiency virus." *New England Journal of Medicine* 317:1125–1135(1987).

Gallo, R. C., M. Robert-Guroff, F. Wong-Stall, et al. "HTLV/LAV and the origin and pathogenesis of AIDS." *International Archives of Allergy and Applied Immunology* 82:471–475(1987).

Ho, D. D., R. J. Pomerantz, and J. C. Kaplan. "Pathogenesis of infection with human immunodeficiency virus." *New England Journal of Medicine* 317:278–286(1987).

Hoff, R., V. P. Berarde, B. J. Weiblen, et al. "Seroprevalence of human immunodeficiency virus among childbearing women. Estimation by testing samples of blood from newborns." *New England Journal of Medicine* 318:525–530(1988).

Konotey-Ahulu, F. I. D. "Clinical epidemiology, not seroepidemiology, is the answer to Africa's AIDS problem." *British Medical Journal* 294: 1593–1594(1987).

Moss, A. R. "Predicting who will progress to AIDS. At least four laboratory predictors available." *British Medical Journal:* 297:1067–1068(1988).

Moss, A. R., P. Bacchetti, D. Osmond, et al. "Seropositivity for HIV and the development of AIDS or AIDS-related condition: three-year follow-up of the San Francisco General Hospital cohort." *British Medical Journal* 296:745–750(1988).

Peterman, T. A., R. L. Stoneburner, J. R. Allen, H. W. Jaffe, and J. W. Curran. "Risk of human immunodeficiency virus transmission from heterosexual adults with transfusion-associated infections." *Journal of the American Medical Association* 295:55–58(1988).

Pyun, K. H., H. D. Ochs, M. T. W. Dufford, and R. J. Wedgwood. "Perinatal infection with human immunodeficiency virus. Specific antibody responses by the neonate." *New England Journal of Medicine* 317:611–614(1987).

Rothenberg, R., M. Woelfel, R. Stoneburner, et al. "Survival with the acquired immunodeficiency syndrome." Experience with 5,833 cases in New York City." *New England Journal of Medicine* 317:1297–1302 (1987).

Schwartz, J. S., P. E. Dans, and B. P. Kinosian. "Human immunodeficiency virus test evaluation, performance, and use. Proposals to make good tests better." *Journal of the American Medical Association* 259:2574–2579(1988).

Ward, J. W., S. D. Holmberg, J. R. Allen, et al. "Transmission of human immunodeficiency virus (HIV) by blood transfusions screened as negative for HIV antibody." *New England Journal of Medicine* 318:473–478(1988).